Leg Ulcers
A practical approach to management

David Negus MA, DM, MCh, FRCS

Teacher in Surgery, University of London, United Medical and Dental Schools of Guy's and St Thomas's Hospitals; Consultant Surgeon, Lewisham and Hither Green Hospitals, London; Membre d'Honneur, Société Française de Phlébologie

with radiological contributions by

Huw Walters FRCR

Consultant Radiologist, King's College Hospital, London

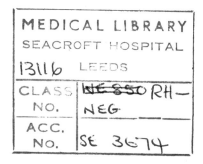
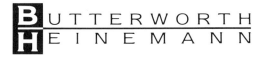

BUTTERWORTH
HEINEMANN

Butterworth–Heinemann Ltd
Halley Court, Jordan Hill, Oxford OX2 8EJ

 PART OF REED INTERNATIONAL P.L.C.

OXFORD LONDON GUILDFORD BOSTON MUNICH NEW DELHI
SINGAPORE SYDNEY TOKYO TORONTO WELLINGTON

First published 1991

© **Butterworth–Heinemann Ltd, 1991**

British Library Cataloguing in Publication Data

Negus, D. (David)
  Leg ulcers.
  1. Man. Legs. Ulcers. Therapy
  I. Title   II. Walters. Huw
  616.5.45

ISBN 0-7506-1034-4

Library of Congress Cataloging-in-Publication Data

Negus, D. (David)
  Leg ulcers: a practical approach to management/
David Negus, with radiological contributions by
Huw Walters.
    p. cm.
  Includes bibliographical references.
  Includes index.
  ISBN 0-7506-1034-4
  1. Leg—Ulcers—Surgery. I. Walters, Huw (Huw
Llewellyn) II. Title.
    [DNLM: 1. Leg Ulcer—therapy. WE 850 N384L]
RD560.N44 1991
617.5′84059—dc20
DNLM/DLC   90-15106

Composition by Genesis Typesetting, Laser Quay, Rochester, Kent
Printed and bound in Great Britain by Courier International Ltd, Tiptree, Essex

Foreword

It is a pleasure and privilege, which I deeply appreciate, to be asked to write a foreword to this excellent little book. David Negus has been a colleague and friend for nearly twenty-five years. He is a general and vascular surgeon, which ensures a good breadth of outlook and experience. For most of his professional life, research on the venous system has been his special interest. He has been deeply involved in many important research projects, notably the early work on the iliac compression syndrome and, later, on methods of early detection and management of deep vein thrombosis. With this background, and much practical experience, he is supremely well qualified to write this book.

Although the main emphasis is on the diagnosis and management of leg ulcers, it is packed with an immense amount of up-to-date general information on the venous system, as a background to his main theme.

Thus in Part I a good and detailed review of anatomy is to be found, followed by interesting sections on the disordered physiology of venous disease and the basic pathology of ulceration. In Part II the real subject of the book, namely leg ulcers, is set out with great understanding and detail. The sections dealing with methods of investigation, differential diagnosis and practical management are particularly outstanding and should be compulsory reading for those who have to deal with these patients.

The profusion of modern methods of so-called non-invasive investigation has been a growth industry over recent years, and the whole subject has become rather confused. In Chapter 7 these methods are all well described, as well as the older and well-tried venography, and a timely attempt has been made to sort out those investigations which are of real practical value in management.

Another time-honoured concept about ulcer dressings is laid to rest in Chapter 9. For generations it has been held that some sort of 'medicated' dressing must be applied to ulcers, and the list of such applications, beloved by manufacturers and hallowed by ancient lore, is simply enormous. The fact that some of these dressings may delay healing, and can sometimes produce chronic skin sensitivity reactions which further complicate the ulcer problem, is rightly stressed here, with much scientific evidence. A simple and safe ulcer dressing regime is described. Stress is also laid on the bacteriology of ulcers and the importance of treating them by parenteral antibiotics, *not* local antibiotics or antiseptics on the dressings.

The differential diagnosis problem in modern practice, where many patients are of an advanced age, is reflected in the increasing incidence of ischaemia and rheumatoid factors in the production of leg ulcers, or complicating venous ulcers which are already present.

Finally, in the last chapter, the whole question of elastic bandages and hosiery is treated in a new and refreshingly scientific manner.

This book should stimulate interest in the widespread and challenging problem of leg ulceration, and help to make the old style 'chronic ulcer clinic' a thing of the past.

F. B. Cockett, MS, FRCS
Consulting Surgeon, St Thomas' Hospital, London

Preface

It is sad but true that there are only four facts about leg ulcers which can be stated without fear of contradiction: they are common, their treatment is time consuming and tedious, they are not life threatening, and most surgeons would prefer someone else to be looking after them.

Many papers have been written on this subject in recent years and most have been incorporated into major textbooks of vascular surgery. It does seem, however, that much of this new work is not easily available to those responsible for the day to day management of leg ulcers and that a considerable communication gap still exists. This book is an attempt to fill that gap. It is intended as a practical handbook, with an emphasis on doing rather than theoretical considerations. This still involves the inclusion of a good deal of the relevant anatomy, physiology, pathology and pharmacology, in order to provide a logical background for the investigation, management and treatment of leg ulcers and the various pathological processes responsible for them. Most previous accounts of leg ulceration have concentrated on venous ulcers and their management and, while these still remain the most common, ischaemia and other causes of ulceration are becoming increasingly frequent and I have tried to place the same emphasis on the diagnosis and management of these as on venous ulceration.

A positive approach to diagnosis and management requires a more pragmatic approach than would be considered acceptable in a conventional textbook. Textbooks which provide a comprehensive review of the many theories of aetiology and discuss conflicting approaches to management may confuse those faced with practical problems, particularly if they are relatively new to the subject. My apology for being dogmatic is therefore a fairly small one.

In works of this sort it is traditional to start with an account of the historical background of the subject. In discussing leg ulceration, this is by no means of merely academic interest. A brief glance at Chapter 1 shows that, until relatively recently, the mainstay of treating leg ulcers was by dressings and compression bandaging. The results of this treatment were, and still are, dismal. Only relatively recently have surgeons become actively involved in treatment, with some encouraging results. Even today, too few surgeons show an interest in the subject, which must inevitably occupy a lowly place in the vascular surgeon's repertoire in comparison to life or limb threatening arterial disorders. This book is therefore intended mainly for surgeons, particularly surgeons in training, for we look to them for future advances. I hope that it will also be read by general practitioners, dermatologists, district nurses and those nurses who run hospital ulcer clinics, and that it will show them that there is more to healing ulcers than changing the type of dressing or antibiotic used and that healing an ulcer is by no means the end of the story. Most venous ulcers can be healed in three months or so, whatever form of dressing is used. A large proportion of these subsequently break down, usually two or three years later. Long-term healing and prevention of recurrence depends on the accurate diagnosis and correction of the underlying vascular abnormality and this often requires some form of surgical treatment. The surgeon faced with this responsibility today can be encouraged by the many recent advances in diagnosis and management, which will help him in his task. By nature the surgeon has to be an optimist, and the management of leg ulcers can now be approached with more optimism than ever before.

I am grateful to a very large number of people who have influenced and helped me over the years. First among these must be my old chief and friend, Frank Cockett, who supervised my early research into the post-thrombotic syndrome and has helped me much since that time. The late Harold Dodd was also a good friend and adviser. Professor Norman Browse has been a continually constructive critic.

I owe very many thanks to Dr Dorothy Vollum; there has been close co-operation between her ulcer clinic and my surgical clinic for many years. I owe most of my knowledge of allergic dermatitis and vasculitic ulceration to her and she has kindly revised my amateur attempts to describe the latter and has provided an appropriate illustration. I am most grateful to Huw Walters for contributing the sections on arteriography and venography. His considerable experience and skill in venography, often a difficult investigation, has proved invaluable in sorting out many complicated venous disorders. Robert Gardiner, Director Medi UK, has given me a great deal of help in writing the chapter on compression hosiery, for which he has also provided illustrations. Dr Zoheir Farid and Dr J. R. Steel have provided much useful information about tropical sores.

Many generations of registrars, house surgeons and technicians have worked hard to care for these patients and I am grateful for their help. Ann Friedgood collected the data for the first ulcer follow-up study and the second is largely the work of Tom Holme, now Senior Surgical Registrar at Ninewells Hospital, Dundee. At Butterworth-Heinemann Geoffrey Smaldon has been an encouraging influence at all times, and his colleagues have been unfailingly helpful and efficient. Peter Cox's ability to produce clear and simple illustrations has been invaluable.

This list would not be complete without mention of a number of nurses: Mrs Cole and Mrs Lloyd, who have looked after my clinics for the past ten years; Mrs Dale, Senior Community Nursing Officer, Midlothian Region of Scotland, and Julia Cornwall, Nursing Sister, Northwick Park Hospital, with whom I have had much useful discussion.

My secretary, Jenny Poole, has kept references and illustrations in good order and the typing has been done by Pauline Carlton with her usual unruffled efficiency.

I am continually grateful to my wife Anne for her patience and help.

D.N.

Contents

Sources of illustrations

Permission to reproduce illustrations from the following authors, publishers and institutions is gratefully acknowledged.

Cover, Figures 3.2, 3.6: The Wellcome Museum of Anatomy, by kind permission of The President and Council of the Royal College of Surgeons of England.
Figure 1.1: The Wellcome Institute Library, London.
Figures 3.1, 3.4, 3.9, 3.11, 4.1, 4.7, 6.2, 6.5, 10.1, 10.12: *Operative Surgery and Management*, edited by J. Keen, Bristol, John Wright & Sons, 1987.
Figure 4.4: H. Dodd, and F. B. Cockett, *The Pathology and Surgery of the Veins of the Lower Limb,* Edinburgh, Churchill Livingstone, 1976.
Figure 4.6: *Surgery of the Veins*, edited by J. J. Bergan and J. S. T. Yao, Orlando, Grune and Stratton, 1983.
Figure 5.5: S. S. Rose ChM, FRCS.
Figure 5.7: *Pathology and Surgery in Clinical Practice,* edited by G. J. Hadfield, M. Hobsley and B. C. Morson, London, Arnold, 1985.
Figures 7.1, 7.2, 7.3, 7.5, 7.6. 7.7, 7.8. 7.9, 7.10, 7.11, 7.12: *Diagnostic Techniques and Assessment of Procedures in Vascular Surgery,* edited by R. M. Greenhalgh, Orlando, Grune and Stratton, 1985.
Figure 8.8: Dr Dorothy Vollum FRCP, Consultant Dermatologist, Lewisham Hospital.
Figures 10.9, 10.10: The late Harold Dodd ChM, FRCS.
Figures 12.1, 12.4, 12.5: R. N. Gardiner, Director, Medi UK Ltd, Hereford.
Figure 12.3: Segar Design, Nottingham.

Part I

Basic principles

Chapter 1

Historical background*

Venous disorders

Although there are references to varicose veins in early Egyptian and Greek writings, the first known mention of leg ulcers is by Hippocrates (460–377 BC)[3], who apparently recognised some relationship between leg ulcers and venous disorders.

A Roman physician, Aurelius Cornelius Celsus (25 BC–AD 50)[4] advised the use of plasters and linen bandages in the treatment of ulcers and also treated varicose veins by avulsion and cauterisation. These procedures were also described by the later Roman physicians Claudius Galen (AD 130–200)[5] and Aetios of Amida (AD 502–574)[6].

During the Dark Ages, those with unsightly and ulcerated legs were denied even simple remedies. Haly, son of Abbas, (d. 994)[7] believed that bandaging varicose legs would reintroduce 'black bile' into the circulation and lead to madness. Avicenna in the tenth century[8] believed that to cure an ulcer was to prevent the efflux of dangerous humours and this widely-held belief persisted until the eighteenth century, when it was expounded by Le Dran in France in 1731[9] and by Heister (but only in elderly patients) in 1739[10]. However, some ligation of varicose veins continued during this period, the reason being 'to intercept the passage of the blood and humour mixed together therewith, flowing to an ulcer seated beneath' (Paré, 1579)[11].

During the seventeenth century the humoral theory gradually began to lose ground and a new confidence was exhibited in the treatment of leg ulcers. Richard Wiseman described a laced stocking in 1676[12] and its use was later recommended by Benjamin Bell (1779)[13]. Wiseman made another significant contribution; he described the formation of a blood coagulum and states that this is due to stagnation 'by reason of dependence of the part or some other pressure on the vessel'. He mentions pregnancy and riding horses as contributory causes.

John Hunter (1775)[14] described the association of thrombosis and phlebitis, both in man after venesection and in horses which had been bled by their ostlers. His specimens illustrate venous and perivenous inflammation, though the prevalence of infection at that time makes it likely that this was bacterial in origin rather than an

---

* Those with a particular interest in the history of medicine should also read the historical sections in Dodd and Cockett's *The Pathology and Surgery of the Veins of the Lower Limb*[1] and in *Diseases of the Veins* by N. L. Browse, K. G. Burnand and M. Lea Thomas[2].

aseptic thrombophlebitis. He also showed interest in leg ulcers and wrote 'the sores of poor people are often in a bad condition from bad living and are often healed by rest in a horizontal position, fresh provisions and warmth in hospitals, and the change is generally very speedy'.

The next century saw significant advances in knowledge of the processes involved in thrombosis. Hewson described a 'coagulable lymph' in 1772[15] and phlebitis and periphlebitic inflammation were described by Carl Rokitansky in 1852[16]. In 1860 Rudolph Virchow[17] described the association between thrombosis in the legs and emboli in the lungs and in subsequent publications he introduced the term 'fibrinogen' and also his famous triad of the causes of thrombosis (stasis, endothelial damage and changes in coagulability). Von Strauch observed venous thrombosis following surgical operation in 1894[18] and this relationship was studied by Cordiér in 1905[19], who found a 2% incidence of phlebitis following abdominal and pelvic operations in a study of 232 cases.

During the eighteenth century it began to be realised that leg ulcers were not necessarily accompanied by visible varicose veins. Many eighteenth century writers, including Bell (1779)[13], Baynton (1797)[20] and Whately (1799)[21] make no reference to varicose veins as a cause of ulceration, although Benjamin Brodie (1846)[22] still held to the varicose theory of ulceration. Baynton introduced paste bandaging and Brodie also used plaster and bandages to heal ulcers and recognised that some dressings caused sensitivity reactions.

A significant contribution to present knowledge was made by John Gay in 1868[23] (Figure 1.1). He described the perforating veins of the calf and ankle, recorded the fact that ulcers could occur in the absence of varicose veins if there had been post-thrombotic damage to the deep veins, and introduced the term 'venous ulcer'. He described clot formation and post-thrombotic recanalisation. His observations were fully supported by those of Spender (1868)[24]. Gay was also the first to describe compression of the left common iliac vein as it passes beneath the right common iliac artery and also correctly described the subfascial course of the proximal short saphenous vein in the upper one-third of the calf which, until recently, has been incorrectly described in most anatomical textbooks.

Gay's work seems to have been overlooked by early twentieth century writers until, in 1916, John Homans[25] introduced the title 'post-phlebitic syndrome'. Homans divided ulcers into those associated with varicose veins of the leg, easily cured by removal of these veins, and post-phlebitic ulcers, 'rapid in development, always intractable to palliative treatment, generally incurable by the removal of varicose veins alone and must be excised to be cured'. Homans described valve destruction by the organisation of thrombus. Later, in 1928[26], he found that nearly all severe post-phlebitic cases had had at some time a 'milk leg' or iliofemoral thrombosis.

In 1928 Franklin[27] published an historical survey of the discovery of valves in veins and this stimulated interst in venous physiology and pathology. In his monograph published in 1931, Turner Warwick[28] reviewed the history of the subject and described the 'bleed back' test which is still used at operation to test the competence of valves in the perforating veins. In 1937 Edwards and Edwards[29] showed that venous thrombosis destroyed valves but was frequently followed by recanalisation. Also in 1937 the use of heparin was first described by Murray and his colleagues[30].

In 1939 Crafoord[31] described the use of heparin in the treatment of post-operative deep vein thrombosis and in 1941 Crafoord and Jorpes[32] used

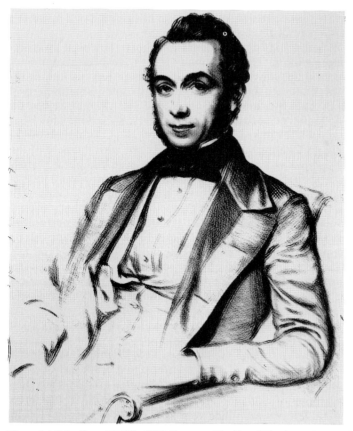

Figure 1.1 John Gay, 1812(3)–1885, Surgeon, The Royal Northern Hospital, London. From the original lithograph of 1853 by T. H. Maguire in the Wellcome Institute Library, London

heparin as a prophylactic agent. In 1950 the use of low doses of heparin for the prevention of deep vein thrombosis was suggested by De Takats[33] and further advances in this method of prophylaxis have been much assisted by advances in phlebography and by the introduction of the isotope-labelled fibrinogen uptake method of detecting deep vein thrombosis. De Takats' work has been continued in numerous studies, of which the largest was the International Multicentre Trial organised by Kakkar (1974)[34].

Clinical phlebography was described by Dos Santos in 1938[35], based on Ratschow's introduction of water soluble X-ray contrast material in 1930[36]. Dos Santos's technique was subsequently used by Gunnar Bauer in Sweden in 1940[37] to study the effect of anticoagulation on deep vein thrombosis and in 1942[38] he undertook an important phlebographic study of the post-thrombotic syndrome. The development, in 1984[39], of low osmolality, non-ionic contrast media, which are virtually non-thrombogenic, has much improved the safety and applicability of phlebography.

In 1960 Hobbs and Davis[40] described the detection of venous thrombi with radioisotopes and this was subsequently validated by comparison with phlebography in two independent clinical studies by Flanc *et al.*[41] and Negus[42] in 1968.

Phlebography and the ^{125}I-fibrinogen uptake technique have stimulated a flood of research into the prevention of deep vein thrombosis.

The ligation of incompetent perforating veins had been practised by some surgeons since Gay's description in 1868, but many must have been discouraged from treating venous ulcers in this way by the difficulty of dissection and finding the offending veins in indurated subcutaneous tissue affected by lipodermatosclerosis. A significant advance was made by Linton of Boston in 1938[43], who described the subfascial ligation of incompetent perforating veins. In 1953 Cockett and Elgin Jones[44] undertook careful cadaver dissections to obtain precise information on the sites of the calf and ankle perforating veins and showed that, with the help of this knowledge, extrafascial ligation was possible. They introduced the phrase 'ankle blow-out syndrome'. A modification of Linton's operation was introduced in 1964 by Harold Dodd[45], who showed that improved skin healing could be obtained by placing the incision for subfascial ligation posteromedially rather than through medial liposclerotic skin. These authors stimulated a wave of interest in perforating vein ligation in the treatment of venous ulceration and between 1961 and 1971 a number of carefully conducted follow-up studies of this operation were reported. Taking these together, over a thousand patients were followed up for between five and nine years, with a success rate of around 90%[46-51]. However in the subsequent ten years, disappointing results in patients with deep venous incompetence as well as perforating vein incompetence have led to a more careful appraisal[52-57] and many surgeons now advise against any attempt at surgical treatment for these patients, relying on elastic compression hosiery alone.

In 1954 Warren and Thayer[58] described the use of the saphenous vein for bypassing a post-thrombotic occlusion of the superficial femoral vein and this operation was further developed by Husni in 1970[59]. Iliac vein occlusion was first similarly treated by femorofemoral bypass by Palma et al. in 1958[60, 61] and these operations have been followed by a number of other ingenious procedures to improve venous function; descriptions can be found in Chapter 10.

At the same time as these advances in diagnosis and treatment, physiological tests of venous function have been developed and are now invaluable in the investigation of the post-thrombotic syndrome and other venous disorders. Venous pressure in the dorsal veins of the foot was first measured by Beecher et al. in 1936[62] and has since been used by many workers[63-67]. Early measurements were made using a saline manometer; the subsequent introduction of the more sophisticated pressure transducer has allowed precise analysis of pressure changes[68].

The introduction of the ultrasonic Doppler-shift velocity meter by Satomura and Kanecko in 1960[69] was the first of the new non-invasive measurement techniques. Venous disorders can now be investigated by a variety of non-invasive methods (described in Chapter 7) which provide an accurate evaluation of venous function without any patient discomfort.

Ischaemic ulceration

As an increasing number of leg ulcers are now ischaemic in origin, this account would be incomplete without a brief mention of the more important milestones in the investigation and treatment of arterial disease.

Carrel[70] is usually credited with the first large-scale experimental series, which demonstrated that arteries could be safely divided and resutured. This was in 1907 and it took a further 40 years before these technqiues were applied to the treatment of patients with atherosclerosis. During this time, it was widely held that, while suture of transected normal arteries was possible, any attempt to perform this procedure in diseased atherosclerotic arteries would be doomed to failure. During this time, therefore, the treatment of peripheral ischaemia was limited to lumbar sympathectomy, first introduced by René Leriche of Strasbourg. The introduction of heparin[30] in 1937 encouraged further attempts at direct arterial surgery and embolectomy was frequently performed in vascular clinics, particularly that of Leriche. One of the surgeons working with René Leriche was J. Cid Dos Santos, who removed some atheromatous intima during the performance of an embolectomy[71]. In spite of this 'mistake', the artery remained patent. Dos Santos and Leriche were encouraged by this success to remove atherosclerotic intima from chronically occluded arteries, and the term 'thrombo-endarterectomy' was applied to this operation[72]. Surgeons around the world were encouraged by this success, and in the 1950s and 1960s the long endarterectomy became the standard procedure for atherosclerotic arterial occlusions. An additional technical advance was Edward's introduction of the patch graft to widen the artery and maintain full flow[73]. Since those pioneering days, endarterectomy has gradually given way to bypass grafting. Kunlin[74] described the use of the reverse saphenous vein graft in 1951, and Hall[75] designed a 'valvulotome' which enabled the use of *in situ* saphenous vein by destruction of its valves. While the saphenous vein was found to be of sufficient diameter to bypass the occluded superficial femoral artery, the aorta and iliac arteries demanded larger diameter tubes and many surgeons used homografts harvested from young patients with healthy arteries who had died from an unrelated disease. Many of these implanted arteries became aneurysmal as a result of an immune rejection reaction and, when synthetic grafts such as crimped Dacron (Terylene)[76] became more easily available, homografts were abandoned.

Other synthetic grafts of relatively recent introduction are the polytetra-fluoroethylene (PTFE) grafts which were originally developed by the Gore Company (Gore-Tex) and introduced by Soyer in 1972[77], the Dardik graft[78] produced by tanning human umbilical cord vein with gluteraldehyde, the bovine carotid artery graft treated by ficin and tanned with dialdehyde starch[79], and the Sparks Mandril[80]. Of these, only the PTFE and Dardik grafts have stood the test of time. Argument continues on their respective merits; Veith has demonstrated long-term patency rates of femoropopliteal PTFE grafts similar to those of autogenous spahenous vein[81], but synthetic grafts are unsatisfactory for the treatment of longer occlusions, requiring anastomosis to the crural vessels.

As in the investigation of venous disorders, the diagnosis and management of peripheral arterial disease has been much assisted by new radiological techniques, particularly digital subtraction angiography, and the non-invasive techniques of colour-coded Duplex scanning and Magnetic Resonance Imaging are now being introduced to major centres of vascular surgery. The simple hand-held Doppler ultrasound apparatus has become an essential tool for the vascular surgeon.

The radiologist is no longer simply a diagnostician; large numbers of patients with arterial stenoses or occlusions less than 10 cm in length are now treated by balloon angioplasty (percutaneous transluminal angioplasty, PTA), and this technique is often successful in treating ischaemic ulceration or relieving rest pain or impending gangrene in elderly patients considered unfit for direct arterial surgery.

In addition to these technical advances, there have been some encouraging developments in the drug treatment of peripheral vascular disease, particularly the introduction of the vasoactive prostaglandins, PGE_1 and PGI_2, and these are described in Chapter 11.

References

1. Dodd, H., Cockett, F. B. *The Pathology and Surgery of the Veins of the Lower Limb*, 2nd edn, Edinburgh, Churchill Livingstone, p. 3, 1976
2. Browse, N. L., Burnand, K. G., Lea Thomas, M. *Diseases of the Veins; Pathology, Diagnosis and Treatment*, London, Edward Arnold, p. 1, 1988
3. Hippocrates. De ulceribus and De carnibus. In *The Genuine Works of Hippocrates* (ed. Adams, F.), London, Sydenham Society, 1849
4. Celsus, A. A. C. *Of Medicine, in Eight Books* (translated by James Grieve; revised by George Futuoge), London, Renshaw, 1838
5. Galen, C. *Ad scripti libri,* Venice, Vincentium Valgressium, 1562, p. 34, quoted by Anning, S. T. in *The Pathology and Surgery of the Veins of the Lower Limb* (eds Dodd, H., Cockett, F. B.), Edinburgh, Churchill Livingstone, p. 4, 1976
6. Aetios of Amida. Translated from the Latin edition of *Cornarius*, 1542, by Ricci, J. V., Philadelphia, Blakeston, 1950
7. Haly filius Abbas. Translated from Arabic into Latin by Michaele of Capella (1523). Quoted by Anning, S. T. in *The Pathology and Surgery of the Veins of the Lower Limb,* 2nd edn. (eds Dodd, H., Cockett, F. B), Edinburgh, Churchill Livingstone, 1976
8. Avicenna. *De ulceribus, Liber IV.* Quoted by Underwood, M. in *A Treatise on Ulcers of the Legs,* London, Matthews, 1783
9. Le Dran, H. F. *Observations de Chirurgie,* Vol. 1, Paris, Osmont, 1731
10. Heister, L. *A General System of Surgery* (Author's preface: Helmstaadt, 1739), London, Whiston, Innys, Davis, Clarke, Mansby, Cox, Whiston, 1748
11. Paré, A. (1579) Quoted by Johnson, T. in *The works of that famous chirurgion Ambrose Parey,* London, 1634
12. Wiseman, R. *Several Chirurgical Treatises,* London, Wilthoe and Knapton, 1676
13. Bell, B. *Treatise on the Theory and Management of Ulcers etc.,* Edinburg, C. Elliot, 1779
14. Hunter, J. Observation on the inflammation of the internal coats of veins (1775). In *The Works of John Hunter* (ed. Palmer, J. I.), London, Longman, Rees, Orme, Green and Longman, pp. 581–586, 1837
15. Hewson, W. *Experimental Enquiries. Part I. An Enquiry into the Properties of Blood,* London, Cadell, 1772
16. Rokitansky, C. *A Manual of Pathological Anatomy* (translated by Gay, G. E.), London, Sydenham Society, p. 336, 1852
17. Virchow, R. *Cellular Pathology as Based upon Physiological and Pathological Histology,* London, Churchill, 1860
18. Von Strauch, N. Über Venenthrombose der Unteren Extremitäten nach Köliotomien bei Beckenhochlagerung und Äthernarkose. *Zentralbl. Gynäkol.* **18**: 304–306, 1894
19. Cordiér, A. N. Phlebitis following abdominal and pelvic operations. *J. A. M. A.* **45**: 1792–1796, 1905
20. Baynton, T. *Descriptive Account of New Method of Treating Old Ulcers of the Legs,* Bristol, Biggs, 1797
21. Whately, T. *Practical Observations on the Cure of Wounds and Ulcers of the Legs Without Rest,* London, Cadell and Davies, 1799
22. Brodie, B. C. *Lectures Illustrative of Various Subjects in Pathology and Surgery,* London, Longmans, p. 158, 1846
23. Gay, J. On varicose disease of the lower extremities and its allied disorders. *Lettsomian Lectures of 1867,* London, Churchill, 1868
24. Spender, J. K. *A Manual of the Pathology and Treatment of Ulcers and Cutaneous Diseases of the Lower Limbs,* London, Churchill, 1868

25. Homans, J. The operative treatment of varicose veins and ulcers, based on a classification of these lesions. *Surg. Gynecol. Obstet.* **22**: 143–158, 1916
26. Homans, J. Thrombophlebitis of the lower extremities. *Ann. Surg.* **87**: 641–651, 1928
27. Franklin, K. J. The valves in veins. An historical survey. *Proc. R. Soc. Med.* (Section of History of Medicine) **21**: 1–33, 1927
28. Warwick, W. T. *The Rational Treatment of Varicose Veins and Varicocele,* London, Faber, 1931
29. Edwards, F. A., Edwards, J. E. The effect of thrombophlebitis on the venous valves. *Surg. Gynecol. Obstet.* **65**: 310–320, 1937
30. Murray, D. W. G., Jaques, L. B., Perrett, T. S., Best, C. H. Heparin and the thrombosis of veins following injury. *Surgery* **2**: 163–187, 1937
31. Crafoord, C. Heparin and post-operative thrombosis. *Acta Chir. Scand.* **82**: 319–335, 1939
32. Crafoord, C., Jorpes, E. Heparin as a prophylactic against thrombosis. *J. A. M. A.* **116**: 2831–2835, 1941
33. De Takats, G. Anticoagulant therapy in surgery. *J. A. M. A.* **142**: 527–534, 1950
34. International Multicentre Trial. Heparin versus dextran in the prevention of deep vein thrombosis. *Lancet* **2**: 118–120, 1974
35. Dos Santos, J. C. La phlébographie directe. Conception, technique, premiers résultats. *J. Int. Chir.* **3**: 625–669, 1938
36. Ratschow, M. Euroselektan in der Vasographie. Unter spezieller Berücksichtigung der Varikographie. *Fortsch. Rontgenstr.* **42**: 37, 1930
37. Bauer, G. A venographic study of thromboembolic patients. *Acta Chir. Scand.* **84**: suppl. 61, 1940
38. Bauer, G. A roentgenological and clinical study of the sequels of thrombosis. *Acta Chir. Scand* **86**: suppl. 74, 1942
39. Lea Thomas, M., Biggs, G. M. Low osmolality contrast media for phlebography. *Int. Angiol.* **3**: 73–76, 1984
40. Hobbs, J. T., Davis, J. W. L. Detection of venous thrombosis with ^{131}I-labelled fibrinogen in the rabbit. *Lancet* **2**: 134–135, 1960
41. Flanc, C., Kakkar, V. V., Clark, M. B. The detection of venous thrombosis of the legs using ^{125}I-labelled fibrinogen. *Br. J. Surg.* **55**: 742–747, 1968
42. Negus, D., Pinto, D. J., Le Quesne, L. P., Brown, N., Chapman, H. ^{125}I-labelled fibrinogen in the diagnosis of deep vein thrombosis and its correlation with phlebography. *Br. J. Surg.* **55**: 835–839, 1968
43. Linton, R. R. The communicating veins of the lower leg and the operative technique for their ligation. *Ann. Surg.* **107**: 582–593, 1938
44. Cockett, F. B., Elgin Jones, D. E. The ankle blow-out syndrome. A new approach to the venous ulcer problem. *Lancet* **1**: 17–23, 1953
45. Dodd, H. The diagnosis and ligation of incompetent perforating veins. *Ann. R. Coll. Surg. Engl.* **34**: 186–196, 1964
46. Burnley, J. J., Krausers Trasser, E. S. Chronic venous insufficiency of the lower extremities. *Surgery* **49**: 48–58, 1961
47. Hansson, L. O. Venous ulcers of the lower limb. *Acta Chir. Scand.* **128**: 269–277, 1964
48. Bertelsen, S., Gammelgaard, A. Surgical treatment of post-thrombotic leg ulcers. *J. Cardiovasc. Surg.* **6**: 452–455, 1965
49. Silver, D., Gleysteen, J. J., Rhodes, G. R., *et al.* Surgical treatment of the refractory post-thrombotic ulcers. *Arch. Surg.* **103**: 554–560, 1971
50. Field, P., Van Boxall, P. The role of the Linton flap procedure on the management of stasis dermatitis and ulceration in the lower limbs. *Surgery* **70**: 920–926, 1971
51. Arnoldi, I. C., Haeger, K. Ulcus cruris venosum – crux medicorum? *Läkartidningen* **64**: 2149–2157, 1967
52. Recek, E. A critical appraisal of the role of ankle perforators for the genesis of venous ulcers in the lower legs. *J. Cardiovasc. Surg.* **12**: 45–49, 1971
53. Burnand, K. G., Lea Thomas, M., O'Donnell, E., *et al.* Relation between post-phlebitic changes in the deep veins and results of surgical treatment of venous ulcers. *Lancet* **1**: 936–938, 1976
54. Kiely, P. E. Surgery should be avoided in patients with deep vein incompetence and without superficial varices. Personal communication, 1982
55. Strandness, D. E., Thiele, D. L. *Selected Topics in Venous Disorders,* New York, Futura, 1981

56. Lumley, J. S. P. Surgical treatment of varicose veins. In *Contemporary Operative Surgery* (ed. Marston A.), London, Northwood Books, 1979
57. Browse, N. L., Burnand, K. G. The causes of venous ulceration. *Lancet* **2**: 243–245, 1982
58. Warren, R., Thayer, T. Transplantation of the saphenous vein for post-phlebitic stasis. *Surgery* **35**: 867–876, 1954
59. Husni, E. A. In situ saphenopopliteal bypass graft for incompetence of the femoral and popliteal veins. *Surg. Gynecol. Obstet.* **130**: 279–284, 1970
60. Palma, E. C., Ricci, F., De Campo, F., Tratamiento de los trastronos post flebiticos mediante anastomosis venosa safenofemoral contro-lateral. *Bull. Soc. Surg. Uruguay* **29**: 135, 1958
61. Palma, E. C., Esperon, R. Vein transplants and grafts in the surgical treatment of the post-phlebitic syndrome. *J. Cardiovasc. Surg.* **1**: 94–107, 1960
62. Beecher, H. K., Field, M. E., Krogh, L. The effect of walking on the venous pressure at the ankle. *Scand. Arch. Physiol.* **73**: 133, 1936
63. Warren, R., White, E. A., Beecher, C. D. Venous pressures in the saphenous system in normal, varicose and post-phlebitic extremities. *Surgery* **26**: 435–445, 1949
64. Pollack, A. A., Wood, E. H. Venous pressure in the saphenous vein of the ankle in man during exercise and changes in posture. *J. Appl. Physiol.* **1**: 649–662, 1949
65. De Camp, P. T., Schramel, R. J., Roy, C. J., Feibleman, N. D., Ward, J. A., Ochsner, A. Ambulatory venous pressure determinations in post-phlebitic and related syndromes. *Surgery* **29**: 44–70, 1951
66. Höjensgard, J. C., Stürup, H. Static and dynamic pressures in superficial and deep veins of the lower extremities in man. *Acta Physiol. Scand.* **27**: 49–67, 1953
67. Arnoldi, C. C. E., Greitz, T., Linderholme, H. Variations in cross-sectional area and pressure in the veins of the normal human leg during rythmical muscular exercise. *Acta Chir. Scand.* **132**: 507–552, 1966
68. Nicolaides, A. N., Hoare, M., Miles, C. R. *et al*. Value of ambulatory venous pressures in the assessment of venous insufficiency. *Vasc. Diagn. Ther.* **3**: 41, 1982
69. Satomura, S., Kanecko, Z. Ultrasonic blood rheograph. Proceedings of the Third International Conference on Medical Electronics, pp. 254–258, 1960
70. Edwards, W. S., Edwards, P. D. *Alexis Carrel, Visionary Surgeon*. Springfield, Illinois, Charles C. Thomas, 1974
71. Dos Santos, J. C. From embolectomy to endarterectomy or the fall of a myth. *J. Cardiovasc. Surg.* **17**: 113–128, 1976
72. Dos Santos, J. C. Sur la désobstruction des thromboses artérielles anciennes. *Mem. Acad. Chir.* **73**: 409–411, 1947
73. Edwards, W. S. Composite reconstruction of the femoral artery with saphenous vein after endarterectomy. *Surg. Gynecol. Obstet.* **111**: 651–653, 1960
74. Kunlin, J. Le traitement de l'ischemie artéritique par la greffe veineuse longue. *Rev. Chir. (Paris)* **70**: 206–235, 1951
75. Hall, K. V. The greater saphenous vein used *in-situ* as an arterial shunt after vein valve extirpation. *Acta Chir. Scand.* **128**: 365–386, 1964
76. Crawford, E. S., De Bakey, M. E., Cooley, D. A., Morris, J. C. Jnr. Use of crimped knitted Dacron grafts in patients with occlusive disease of the aorta and of the iliac, femoral and popliteal arteries. In *Fundamentals of Vascular Grafting* (eds. Wesolowska, S. A. and Dennis, C.), New York, McGraw Hill, pp. 356–366, 1963
77. Soyer, T., Lempinen, M., Cooper, P. *et al*. A new venous prosthesis. *Surgery* **72**: 864–872, 1972
78. Dardik, H., Ibrahim, I. M., Sussman, B. *et al*. Gluteraldehyde-stabilised umbilical vein prosthesis for revascularisation of the legs: three year results by life table analysis. *Am. J. Surg.* **138**: 234–237, 1979
79. Rosenberg, N., Goughrna, E. R. C., Henderson, J. *et al*. The use of segmental arterial implants prepared by enzymatic modification of heterologous blood vessels. *Surg. Forum* **6**: 242–246, 1956
80. Sparks, C. H. Silicon mandril method for growing reinforced autogenous femoro-popliteal artery grafts in-situ. *Ann. Surg.* **177**: 293–300, 1973
81. Veith, F. J. Vein and PTFE bypasses to infrapopliteal arteries. In *Vascular Surgical Techniques* (ed. Greenhalgh, R. M.), London, Butterworths, pp. 199–211, 1984

Chapter 2

The extent of the problem

The scarcity of epidemiological studies on the incidence of leg ulceration probably reflects a general lack of interest in a chronic, non-fatal condition which mainly affects the elderly. Studies in Bohemia and Switzerland have suggested that venous ulceration affects 1% of the population[1,2]. Few UK studies have been undertaken; in 1931 Wright[3] suggested a prevalence of 0.5% and in 1951 Boyd et al.[4] suggested a similar figure, but these authors based their numbers on estimates. A survey conducted in Tecumseh, Michigan, USA[5] found no ulcers in those aged 20–29, but 0.6% in men and 2.1% in women aged between 60 and 69 years. In West Germany, 4530 randomly selected individuals were examined in Tubingen[6] in 1981. Ulcers were found in 2% of women and 3% of men. Maffeii et al.[7] published data on 1755 Brazilian patients over the age of 15. Active or healed ulcers were found in 3.6% with 2.3% of men and 4% of women suffering from the condition. Moffatt and his colleagues[8] found 21 patients with leg ulcers in a population of 7500 (0.28%). The mean age of the ulcer patients was 78 (52–91) years and the average duration of the ulcer was 21 months. These authors estimate a total of 150 000 ulcer patients in the UK, with a cost of £2500 per ulcer, per patient, per year.

In a small study based on patients in a group practice in Edinburgh, Mrs Dale, a senior community nurse, and her co-workers[9] estimated that 1% of adults suffered from chronic leg ulcers, but in the much larger Lothian and Forth Valley Leg Ulcer Study[10], based on a postal survey in two health board areas in Scotland, with a population of about one million, 1477 patients with chronic leg ulcers were identified, an incidence of 1.48/1000 population. The Lothian and Forth Valley Leg Ulcer investigators also demonstrated that most patients suffering from leg ulcers were women and that the condition was common in the elderly, the median age of the men being 67 years (range 22–96) and of the women 74 years (range 21–100), but their survey may not have been complete because they were unable to know what proportion of patients failed to report ulceration to their doctors. It was not possible to identify the cause of ulceration in every patient included in the Lothian and Forth Valley study but, in a smaller study of 600 patients with leg ulcers from this population, Doppler ultrasound examination of 827 ulcerated legs showed evidence of peripheral arterial insufficiency in 176 (21.3%)[11]. Ankle:brachial pressure ratio was less than 0.7 in half of these patients. In a similar study of 357 patients with 425 leg ulcers, in a population of approximately 200 000 in North London, Cornwall and Lewis (1983)[12] found that 80% had some evidence of venous disease and that this was combined with arterial disease in nearly one-third.

In the Lothian and Forth Valley Leg Ulcer Study, patients with rheumatoid disease and diabetes were found to have a greater incidence of leg ulceration than the unaffected population[13]. However, no relationship was found between leg ulceration and hypertension.

The heavy workload imposed on nurses in dressing ulcers has been demonstrated by the Lothian and Forth Valley study[14]. It was found that 71% of 500 patients currently being treated for leg ulceration were treated in their own homes and that this necessitated an average number of three visits per week per patient. Each visit took between 34 and 46 minutes. District nurses were found to be using a wide variety of empirical treatments, paste bandaging being that most frequently used, probably because it had the advantage of reducing the number of visits required.

This study also demonstrated the long-term ineffectiveness of such conservative treatment[10]; most patients had histories of intermittent ulceration longer than 10 years. The duration of ulceration was similarly recorded in 77 patients with 109 ulcerated legs referred to the Lewisham Hospital Vascular Surgical Clinic[15]. These patients had suffered from leg ulcers, usually intermittently, for periods ranging from a few months to 50 years, with a mean of 16.6 years. These patients came from a well-doctored area, and all had been treated by conventional methods before referral to hospital (Table 2.1).

Table 2.1 Treatment of 77 patients before referral to the Lewisham vein clinic

Previous treatment	Patients
Elastic compression and dressings	48
Saphenous ligation and stripping	12
Perforating vein ligation	4
Injection sclerotherapy	6
Injection sclerotherapy + surgery	7
All previous treatments	77

A recent study from Northwick Park Hospital has shown a 46% ulcer recurrence rate in 109 patients treated conservatively by compression hosiery, after initial healing[16]. These poor results indicate that elastic compression is unlikely to produce good long-term results and a more radical approach is required in order to correct the underlying vascular disorder and to prevent ulcer recurrence.

The Lothian and Forth Valley Leg Ulcer Study is the most comprehensive ever undertaken in the UK and has been invaluable in emphasising the large numbers of patients suffering from leg ulceration, the importance of examining patients for arterial as well as for venous insufficiency and the heavy workload that leg ulcers impose on nursing services. It is the main purpose of this book to show that a positive approach to diagnosis and treatment can improve long-term results with a potential reduction in the workload involved.

References

1. Bobek, K., Cajzl, L., Cepelák V., Slaisova, V., Opatzny, K., Barkel, R. Étude de la fréquence des maladies phlébologiques et de l'influence de quelques facteurs étiologiques. *Phlébologie* **19**: 217–230, 1966

2. Widmer, L. K. *Peripheral Venous Disorders; Prevalence and Sociomedical Importance,* Bern, Hans Huber, 1978
3. Wright, A. D. The treatment of indolent ulcer of the leg. *Lancet* **1**: 457–460, 1931
4. Boyd, A. M., Jepson, R. P., Ratcliffe, R. H., Rose, S. S. The logical management of ulcers of the legs. *Angiology* **3**: 207–215, 1952
5. Coon, W. W., Willis, P. W., Keller, J. B. Venous thromboembolism and other venous disease in the Tecumseh Community Health Study. *Circulation* **48**: 839–846, 1973
6. Fischer, H. (Hrsg.) *Venenleiden – Eine repräsentative Untersuchung in Bundesrepublik Deutschland,* Munchen, Urban and Schwarzenberg, 1981
7. Maffeii, F. H., Magaldi, C., Pinho, S. Z., *et al.* Varicose veins and chronic venous insufficiency in Brazil: prevalence among 1755 inhabitants of a country town. *Int. J. Epidemiol.* **15**: 210–217, 1986
8. Moffatt, C., Wright, D. D., Besley, D., McCollum, C., Greenhalgh, R. M. A new approach to chronic venous ulcers in the community. *Br. J. Surg.* **76**: 418, 1989
9. Dale, J. J., Callam, M. J., Ruckley, C. V., Harper, D. R., Berry, P. N. Chronic ulcers of the leg: a study of prevalence in a Scottish community. *Health Bull.* **41**: 310–314, 1983
10. Callam, M. J., Harper, D. R., Dale, J. J., Ruckley, C. V. Chronic ulcer of the leg: clinical history. *Br. Med. J.* **294**: 1389–1391, 1987
11. Callam, M. J., Harper, D. R., Dale, J. J., Ruckley, C. V. Arterial disease in chronic leg ulceration: an underestimated hazard? Lothian and Forth Valley Leg Ulcer Study. *Br. Med. J.* **294**: 929–931, 1987
12. Cornwall, J. V., Lewis, J. D. Leg ulcer revisited. *Br. J. Surg.* **70**: 681, 1983
13. Callam, M. J., Ruckley, C. V., Dale, J. J., Harper, D. R. Chronic leg ulcer. The incidence of associated non-venous disorders. In *Phlebology '85* (eds Negus, D., Jantet, G.), London, Libbey, pp. 542–543, 1986
14. Dale, J. J., Callam, M. J., Harper, D. R., Ruckley, C. V. Chronic leg ulcers. The role of the district nurse. In *Phlebology '85* (eds Negus, D., Jantet, G.), London, Libbey, pp. 621–623, 1986
15. Negus, D., Friedgood, A. The effective management of venous ulceration. *Br. J. Surg.* **70**: 623–627, 1983
16. Cornwall, J. V., Dove, C. J., Chadwick, S. J. D., Lewis, J. D. Leg ulcers resurrected; a 7-year follow-up. Paper read to Venous Forum meeting, Manchester, May 1989

Chapter 3

The anatomy of the veins of the lower limb

A thorough knowledge of the anatomy of the veins of the lower limb is essential for the surgical correction of those abnormalities which underlie venous ulceration. In this review features important to the diagnosis and management of venous disorders have been emphasised.

Histological features

The walls of veins are similar to those of arteries, being composed of three coats: an inner endothelium, a muscular media and an outer fibrous adventitia[1]. However they differ from arteries in a number of important details. The endothelium of the *intima*, unlike that of arteries, secretes Factor XIII, prostacyclins and fibrinolytic activator. Recurrent spontaneous thrombosis occurs in patients with an inherited lack of vein wall activator[2]. The *media* consists of collagen and elastin fibres and non-striated muscle fibres arranged circularly. The elastin fibres are in a smaller proportion than in arterial walls. The muscle fibres are most well developed in the superficial veins, and their contraction is controlled by post-ganglionic adrenergic sympathetic nerve fibres. By contrast, the media of the deep veins contains relatively little muscle and these veins act mainly as passive blood conduits. The *adventitia* consists of areolar tissue with longitudinal elastic fibres. In the largest veins, it is very much thicker than the tunica media and contains longitudinal muscle fibres.

Most veins contain bicuspid valves which direct flow proximally and from the superficial to the deep veins. Valves consist of collagen fibres covered by a thin layer of endothelium and are stronger than the vein wall[3]. Valves are most numerous in the deep veins of the calf and are fewer in the popliteal and femoral veins. The iliac veins are usually valveless[4]. The long saphenous vein contains 3–7 valves[5] and each direct calf perforating vein contains one valve.

Anatomy

The venous drainage of the lower limb is divided into the superficial and deep systems, the drainage areas of which are separated by the deep fascia. Thus the superficial veins, the long and short saphenous veins and tributaries of the perforating veins, drain the skin and subcutaneous fat (the so-called superficial fascia) and the deep veins are responsible for venous return from muscle and other structures deep to the deep fascia. The volume of venous blood passing through the deep system far exceeds that through the superficial; the function of the latter being mainly in temperature regulation. The superficial veins communicate with the deep at the saphenopopliteal and the saphenofemoral junctions and, by way of the perforating veins, through defects in the deep fascia.

Superficial veins

These are the long and short saphenous veins and the tributaries of the perforating veins. The *long saphenous vein* arises from the medial end of the dorsal venous arch of the foot (see Figure 3.3), then passes in front of the medial malleolus and along the medial surface of the leg, enclosed in its own fascial sheath in the superficial fascia[6]. The long saphenous vein lies rather posteriorly at knee level and then passes up the thigh and through the foramen ovale in the femoral triangle to join the common femoral vein. It crosses the superficial external pudendal artery at the lower border of the foramen ovale.

The anatomy of the long saphenous vein and its important tributaries can easily be remembered by thinking of two tridents, or three-part pronged forks, one in the thigh and one just below the knee (Figure 3.1). In the groin the important tributaries are the anterolateral and posteromedial veins of the thigh. Smaller tributaries are the superficial and deep external pudendal veins, and the superficial epigastric and circumflex iliac veins. Just below the knee the anterior and posterior prongs of the trident are the anterior vein of the leg and the posterior arch vein. The important medial calf direct perforating veins communicate with the posterior arch vein (first accurately observed and drawn by Leonardo da Vinci) and *not* directly with the long saphenous vein.

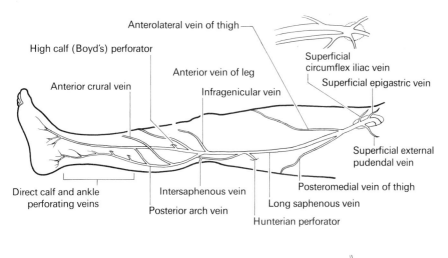

Figure 3.1 The long saphenous vein and its tributaries. Insets: duplication of the long saphenous vein (upper); aberrant superficial external pudendal artery (lower)

The tributaries of the long saphenous vein commonly become varicose; the saphenous vein itself is only occasionally dilated and varicose in the lower leg. The long saphenous vein is accompanied by the saphenous nerve, which is closely applied to the vein in the lower one-third of the calf, where it may be damaged by the passage of a vein stripper (Figure 3.2).

It may seem unnecessary to emphasise that the long saphenous vein lies *in front* of the medial malleolus. The posterior tibial artery passes behind this bony landmark. Failure to remember this very elementary anatomical point has resulted in the femoral artery being stripped on more than one occasion. The long saphenous vein is occasionally duplicated, either in part or the whole of its course. It is also sometimes crossed by the superficial external pudendal artery, instead of passing superficial (anterior) to it. The surgeon must be aware of these anatomical abnormalities if he is to dissect safely and effectively in this area (see Figure 3.1).

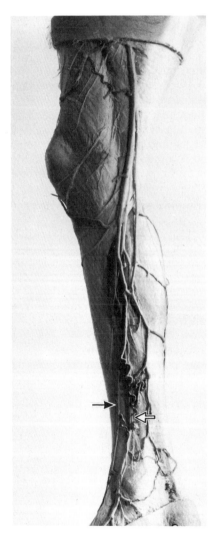

Figure 3.2 The saphenous nerve (white arrow) becomes more closely applied to the long saphenous vein (black arrow) in the lower leg and ankle, where it is more at risk of damage by vein stripping

The dorsal venous arch of the foot communicates with the plantar veins by way of four perforating veins which pass between the metatarsals (Figure 3.3). This apparently unimportant anatomical feature may be to some extent responsible for recurrent venous ulceration and should therefore be remembered.

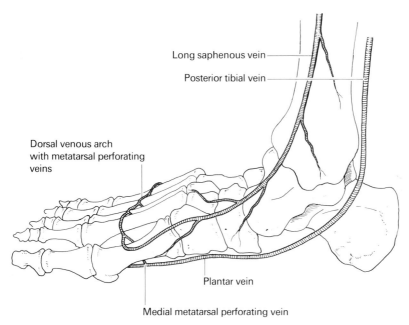

Figure 3.3 The four metatarsal communicating veins join the superficial system (dorsal venous arch) to the deep system of veins (plantar veins) in the foot

The *short saphenous vein* starts at the lateral end of the dorsal venous arch of the foot and passes behind the lateral malleolus to join the popliteal vein in the popliteal fossa. This termination is very variable (Figure 3.4). The high termination occurs in 33% of cases[7]; in this variation the short saphenous vein passes up the posterior surface of the thigh (persistent post-axial vein) and either joins the long saphenous vein or terminates in muscle veins. The low termination occurs in about 9%; the short saphenous vein then joining gastrocnemius veins in the calf.

It is important to realise that the short saphenous vein perforates the deep fascia in the lower or medial third of the calf and lies deep to the deep fascia, between the bellies of gastrocnemius, until it joins the popliteal vein in the popliteal fossa. This feature of the short saphenous vein is described incorrectly in most anatomical textbooks and failure to appreciate this point results in many inadequate operations. The description of the external (short) saphenous vein in the 1897 (14th) edition of *Gray's Anatomy*[8] is accompanied by the following footnote 'Mr. Gay calls attention to the fact that the external saphenous vein often (he says invariably) penetrates the fascia at or about the point where the tendon of the Gastrocnemius commences, and runs below the fascia in the rest of its course, or sometimes among the muscular fibres, to join the popliteal vein. See Gay on *Varicose Disease of the Lower Extremities*, p. 24, where there is also a careful and

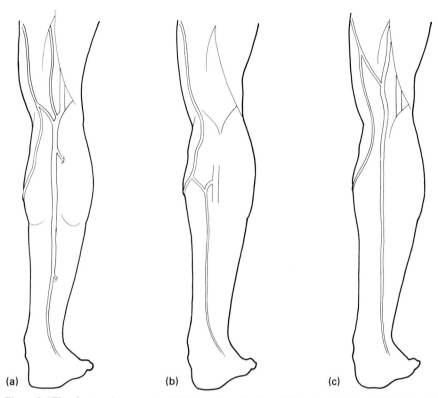

Figure 3.4 The short saphenous vein. (a) Normal termination; (b) low termination; (c) high termination

elaborate description of the branches of the saphena veins.' The same footnote appears in an American edition 'revised' from the 15th English edition (an original copy of this edition has proved impossible to find) but this footnote has disappeared from the 16th and all subsequent editions of *Gray's Anatomy*. As in other aspects of phlebology, Gay appears to have been ahead of his time, and was first grudgingly acknowledged and subsequently ignored by his successors.

The long and short saphenous veins have relatively thick muscle coats, but the walls of their tributaries are thin and more likely to dilate and become varicose.

The *perforating veins* are those veins, other than the long and short saphenous, which penetrate the deep fascia, passing from superficial to deep. Between 50 and 100 unimportant indirect perforating veins enter the muscles before joining the deep veins. These are not normally important to calf muscle pump function, but may dilate and become haemodynamically significant following deep vein thrombosis, recanalisation and reflux. Clinically much more important are the direct perforating veins of the lower half of the leg and ankle, two or three on the medial surface and one or two laterally (Figure 3.5a,b). The medial direct perforating veins communicate with the posterior arch vein, *not* the long saphenous vein itself, and the lateral perforating veins communicate with tributaries of the short saphenous vein. Each perforating vein contains a valve which directs blood from superficial to deep[9]. An easy way to remember their positions is that the

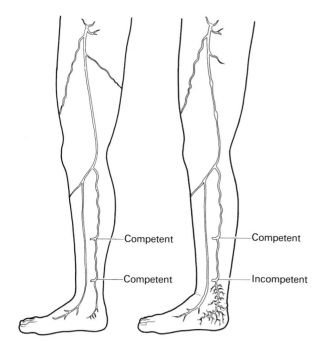

Figure 3.5 The medial direct perforating veins of the calf and ankle. These are usually found in the following sites: I, behind the medial malleolus; II, 8–10 cm above the malleolus; III, 12–15 cm above the malleolus

lowest lies behind the medial malleolus, the next a hand's-breadth above this, and the most proximal another hand's-breadth higher (Cockett's hand's-breadth rule).

The direct calf and ankle perforating veins drain the skin over the medial and lateral malleoli by networks of venules and small veins, the so-called corona phlebectatica. These drain the ulcer bearing areas of the ankle (Figure 3.5 and 3.6). The medial and lateral ankle skin is not directly drained by either the long or short saphenous vein. The long saphenous vein does however communicate with the medial perforating veins through two or three tributaries which can be seen in Figure 3.6 and the distal long saphenous vein also communicates with the plantar veins through the dorsal venous arch of the foot and the transmetatarsal veins. The malleolar venous network ('corona phlebectatica') therefore communicates with the deep system by two routes: directly to the posterior tibial vein through the calf perforating veins and indirectly through the plantar veins by way of the dorsal venous arch. Incompetence of a perforating vein valve results in high pressure in, and dilatation of, the malleolar venules, which results in the ankle venous flare (see Figure 4.5). Perforating vein incompetence and an ankle flare is a common precursor of venous ulceration; other, more proximal, perforating veins are less often incompetent, and are usually related to primary varicose veins.

The hunterian perforators form communications between the long saphenous vein in the lower third of the thigh and the superficial femoral vein in the subsartorial ('Hunter's') canal. Peroperative retrograde saphenography in a series of 60 patients showed at least one hunterian perforator in 87% of 80 saphenograms[10]. Seventy per cent of incompetent thigh perforating veins are found

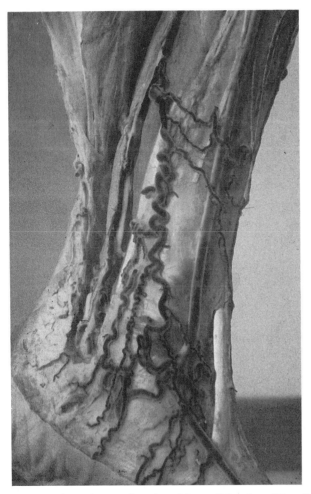

Figure 3.6 Corrosion cast dissection of the medial surface of the calf showing dilated veins of the 'corona phlebectatica' communicating with the posterior tibial vein through an incompetent perforating vein. Note that a number of venules cross the long saphenous vein without communicating with it but there are two communications below the medial malleolus. (Anatomy Museum, Royal College of Surgeons of England)

in the region of the adductor canal[11] and their incompetence is a common cause of recurrent varicose veins of the long saphenous vein following saphenofemoral ligation without stripping[12]. Other, less common, perforating veins are Boyd's perforator, which joins the long saphenous to the posterior tibial vein on the medial surface of the upper calf at the level of the tibial tubercle, and occasionally a similar perforating vein is found on the lateral surface of the upper calf.

Deep veins

The deep veins of the lower leg are the paired venae comitantes of the anterior and posterior tibial and the peroneal arteries, the gastrocnemius veins and the soleus venous arcades. These all join to form the popliteal vein which receives the short saphenous vein. The main calf veins are profusely valved but the soleus arcades dilate into large valveless sinusoids. These important vessels, with a total capacity of about 140 ml, act as reservoirs or ventricles for the calf muscle pump. They are a common site of thrombus initiation.

The calf and ankle direct perforating veins penetrate the deep fascia to join the posterior tibial vein medially and the peroneal vein laterally.

Contraction of the calf muscles, enclosed in their tight fascial sheath, forces blood proximally, reflux being prevented by the numerous valves; during relaxation of the calf muscles blood passes from superficial to deep along the direct perforating veins.

The popliteal vein becomes the superficial femoral vein in the lower thigh. This large vein only contains two or three valves and has few tributaries apart from the hunterian perforator, some muscle veins and the profunda femoris vein, which joins it to form the common femoral vein. The common femoral vein receives the termination of the long saphenous vein and often also a deep pudendal branch. The common femoral vein becomes the external iliac vein at the inguinal ligament and this in turn becomes the common iliac vein after receiving the internal iliac vein at the level of the sacroiliac joint. The iliac veins are usually valveless; in 200 cadaver dissections, valves were only found in 54[4].

The iliac veins and the iliac compression syndrome

It has long been recognised that iliac venous thrombosis affects the left leg more commonly than the right. In 1784 White[13] noticed that the left leg alone was affected by 'white leg of pregnancy' in 7 out of 9 women and this observation was confirmed by two of his contemporaries. At the time white leg of pregnancy was thought to be due to the accumulation of milky lymph in the leg and the left leg preponderance was attributed to the fact that most women were delivered lying on their left side. The left-sided predominance of iliac venous thrombosis was later noticed by Welch (1887)[14] and by Aschoff (1924)[15] and compression of the left common iliac vein was described by John Gay in 1867[16]. This phenomenon has been confirmed in several other series which are shown in Table 3.1.

Post-thrombotic stenosis of the common iliac vein often follows acute thrombosis and is also more common on the left side than the right. A series of 57 patients with post-thrombotic iliac stenosis or occlusion investigated at St Thomas's Hospital in 1967 showed a 70% left-sided incidence[4].

Table 3.1 The incidence of iliofemoral venous thrombosis

Date	Author	Total cases	Incidence (%)		
			Left	Right	Bilateral
1784	White[13]	9	65	35	
1940	Barker et al.[23]	210	72	28	
1943	Ehrich and Krumbhaar[19]	16	50	18.7	31.3
1967	Negus[4]	88	53.5	27	19.5
1967	Mavor and Galloway[24]	38	75.3	24.7	

Some degree of anteroposterior narrowing of the termination of the left common iliac vein, with an increase in the lateral diameter, is common. Iliac venograms, performed in 54 patients with no previous history of deep vein thrombosis and essentially normal veins, showed a partially translucent area at the termination of the left common iliac vein (Figure 3.7). The diameter of the common iliac veins was also investigated by preparing corrosion casts of the iliac vessels in nine cadavers. There was marked flattening of the termination of the left common iliac vein in all but one.

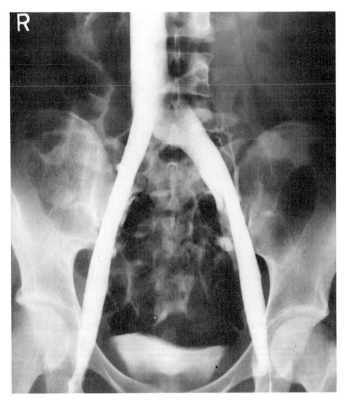

Figure 3.7 Venogram of normal iliac veins and inferior vena cava showing widening and translucency of the termination of the left common iliac vein as it crosses the body of the 5th lumbar vertebra and is crossed by the right common iliac artery

Compression of the left common iliac vein between the convexity of the lumbosacral spine and the overlying right common iliac artery can best be understood by considering the embryology of the iliac veins and inferior vena cava. The lower part of the embryo body is initially drained by the posterior cardinal vein. During the 5th to 7th weeks of embryonic life, a number of additional veins develop: the subcardinal veins which mainly drain the kidneys, the sacrocardinal veins which mainly drain the extremities and the supracardinal veins which form the intercostal veins and take over the function of the posterior cardinal veins (Figure 3.8)[17]. The subcardinal veins communicate at the level of the renal veins

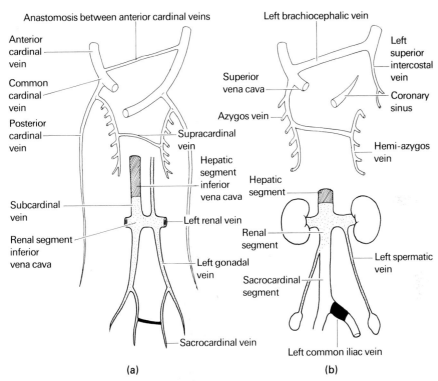

Figure 3.8 Diagrams showing the development of the inferior vena cava, the azygos systems and the superior vena cava. (a) Seventh week of intrauterine life. Note the anastomoses which have formed between the subcardinal, the supracardinal, the sacrocardinal and the anterior cardinal veins. (b) The venous system at birth. Note that the left common iliac vein is formed from the communication between the two sacrocardinal veins

and the left subcardinal vein then develops into the left gonadal vein, the inferior vena cava being formed by fusion of the right subcardinal vein and the right sacrocardinal vein. The left common iliac vein therefore joins the inferior vena cava at almost a right angle (see Figure 3.7), the confluence of the common iliac veins with the inferior vena cava is sometimes illustrated as a Y; this is quite inaccurate.

In passing from left to right to join the inferior vena cava, the left common iliac vein has to traverse the forward prominence of the lumbosacral vertebrae. At the same time it is crossed by the right common iliac artery and these two factors seem responsible for anteroposterior flattening and lateral widening of the termination of the left common iliac vein (Figure 3.9).

Band formation

Bands or spurs joining anterior and posterior walls of the left common iliac vein are not uncommon and appear to be related to extreme degrees of compression of the vein at this point. A typical band is illustrated in Figure 3.10. Bands were found in 14 of 100 dissections performed at St Thomas's Hospital[4] and variations in these are illustrated in Figure 3.11. Lateral bands were found in 6 cases, a central single or double band in 6 cases and almost complete occlusion of the lumen of the vein in 2

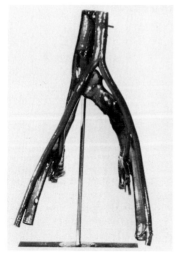

Figure 3.9 Cadaver corrosion cast of the aorta, inferior vena cava and iliac vessels after removal of surrounding soft tissues. Widening and flattening of the termination of the left common iliac vein is clearly seen at the point where it is crossed by the right common iliac artery

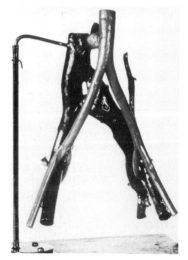

Figure 3.10 Corrosion cast prepared in the same way as that in Figure 3.9. This has been photographed slightly obliquely in order to demonstrate the filling defect at the termination of the left common iliac vein. In life this contained a fibrous 'band'

(a) Lateral flap

(b) Central band

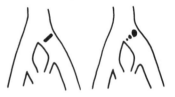

(c) Almost complete occlusion

Figure 3.11 The variety of bands found in 100 dissections of the iliac veins and inferior vena cava

cases. No band was found with any other part of the iliac veins or the inferior vena cava. Histologically these bands consist of fibrous tissue and smooth muscle with a surface of normal endothelium. These bands or spurs were first described by McMurrich in 1906[18] and subsequently by Ehrich and Krumbhaar in 1943[19] and May and Thurner in 1957[20]. Including the author's series, a total of 960 dissections have demonstrated spur formation at the junction of the left common iliac vein and the inferior vena cava in a mean of 22.2%[21] (Table 3.2). There is no histological support for the view that bands originate from an organised thrombus or embolus and they would appear to be developmental and related to compression of the common iliac vein.

There is little doubt that compression of the left common iliac vein and band formation are responsible for the predominantly left-sided incidence of iliofemoral venous thrombosis. The same anatomical anomalies are also responsible for the difficulty in performing left common iliac thrombectomy with a balloon catheter, which often cannot be passed into the inferior vena cava, and also for the failure of this segment of vein to recanalise, resulting in permanent venous occlusion and

Table 3.2 Bands at the mouth of the left common iliac vein

Date	Author	Dissections	Incidence of bands (%)
1906	McMurrich[18]	31	32.3
1943	Ehrich and Krumbhaar[19]	399	23.8
1957	May and Thurner[20]	430	18.6
1968	Negus[21]	100	14.0
	Total	960	Mean 22.2

obstruction to blood flow. This phenomenon has been called the iliac compression syndrome[22]. Many patients with post-thrombotic iliac vein occlusion develop adequate collaterals which compensate for the main vessel obstruction. The pattern of these collaterals is illustrated in Figure 3.12.

Congenital abnormalities of the inferior vena cava include paired cavae, a left-sided cava (persistence of the left subcardinal vein), and occasionally complete absence of the inferior vena cava, blood reaching the heart from the lower limbs by way of the azygos and hemiazygos systems.

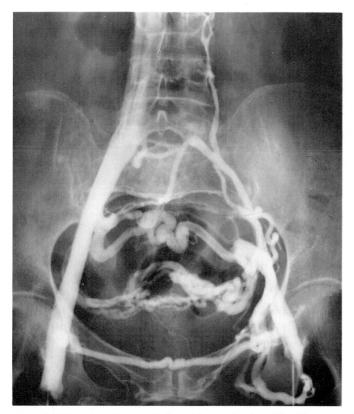

Figure 3.12 Post-thrombotic occlusion of the termination of the left common iliac vein. The following collateral veins can be clearly seen: pudendal, uterine, presacral and the ascending lumbar vein

References

1. Williams, P. L., Warwick, R. (eds) *Gray's Anatomy,* 36th edition, Edinburgh, Churchill Livingstone, 1980
2. Nillson, I.M., Isaacson, S. New aspects of the pathogenesis of thromboembolism. In *Papers in Surgery II* (ed. Allgower, M.), Basel, Karger, p. 46, 1973
3. Ackroyd, J. S., Patterson, M., Browse, N. L. A study of the mechanical properties of fresh and preserved femoral vein wall and valve cusps. *Br. J. Surg* **72**: 117–119, 1985
4. Negus, D. The sequelae of venous thrombosis in the lower limb. *DM Thesis,* University of Oxford, 1967
5. Negus, D. The surgical anatomy of the veins. In *The Pathology and Surgery of the Veins of the Lower Limb,* 2nd edn (eds Dodd, H., Cockett, F. B.), Edinburgh, Churchill Livingstone, p. 35, 1976
6. Papadopoulos, N. J., Sherif, M. F., Albert, E. N. A fascial canal for the great saphenous vein: gross and anatomical observations. *J. Anat.* **132**: 321–329, 1981
7. Kosinski, C. *J. Anat.* London 1926 **60**: 131 quoted in *The Pathology and Surgery of the Veins of the Lower Limb,* 2nd edn (eds Dodd, H. and Cockett, F. B.), Edinburgh, Churchill Livingstone, p. 27, 1976
8. *Gray's Anatomy,* 14th edn, London, Longmans Green, p. 689, 1897
9. Thompson, H. The surgical anatomy of the superficial and perforating veins of the lower limbs. *Ann. R. Coll. Surg. Engl.* **61**: 198–205, 1979
10. Sutton, R., Darke, S. G. Should the long saphenous vein be stripped? A study of per-operative retrograde saphenography. In *Phlebology '85* (eds Negus, D., Jantet, G.), London, Libbey, pp. 196–199, 1986
11. Papadakis, K., Christodoulou, C., Christopoulous, D. *et al.* Number and anatomical distribution of incompetent thigh perforating veins. *Br. J. Surg.* **76**: 581–584, 1989
12. Munn, S. R., Morton, J. B., Macbeth, W. A. A. G., McLeish, A. R. To strip or not to strip the long saphenous vein? A varicose vein trial. *Br. J. Surg.* **68**: 426–428, 1981
13. White, C. *An Inquiry into the Nature and Cause of the Swelling in One or Both of the Lower Extremities, Which Sometimes Happens to Lying-in Women,* Warrington, 1784
14. Welch, W. H. (1887) quoted by Welch, W. H. In *A System of Medicine* (ed. C. Allbutt), London, Macmillan, p. 155, 1899
15. Aschoff, L. *Lecture Notes on Pathology,* New York, Hoeber, 1924
16. Gay, J. On the varicose disease of the lower extremities. *Lettsomian Lectures of 1867,* London, Churchill, 1868
17. Langman, J. *Medical Embryology,* Baltimore, Williams and Wilkins, 1981
18. McMurrich, J. P. The valves of the iliac vein. *Br. Med. J.* **2**: 1699–1700, 1906
19. Ehrich, W. E., Krumbhaar, E. B. A frequent obstructive anomaly of the mouth of the left common iliac vein. *Am. Heart J.* **26**: 737–750, 1943
20. May, R., Thurner, J. The cause of the predominantly sinistral occurrence of thrombosis of the pelvic veins. *Angiology* **8**: 419–427, 1957
21. Negus, D., Fletcher, E. W. L., Cockett, F. B., Lea Thomas, M. Compression and band formation at the mouth of the left common iliac vein. *Br. J. Surg.* **55**: 369–374, 1968
22. Cockett, F. B., Lea Thomas, M. The iliac compression syndrome. *Br. J. Surg.* **52**: 816–821, 1965
23. Barker, N. W., Nygaard, K. K., Walters, W., Priestley, J. T. A statistical study of postoperative venous thrombosis. IV Location of thrombus. *Mayo Clin. Proc.* **16**: 33–37, 1941
24. Mavor, G. E., Galloway, J. M. D. The ilio-femoral venous segment as a source of pulmonary embolism. *Lancet* **1**: 871–874, 1967

Chapter 4

Venous return from the lower limb muscle pumps: normal and disordered function

The veins are the 'capacitance vessels', containing about two-thirds of the total circulating blood volume. Local changes in blood volume are controlled by changes in venous tone mediated by the sympathetic system. The most important function of the superficial veins of the lower limb, as elsewhere in the body, is thermoregulation. Venoconstriction is effected by adrenergic sympathetic nerve endings, and sympathetic stimulation by emotion or pain, or during exercise, also results in superficial vasoconstriction. The deep veins have less powerful muscle coats and mainly act as passive blood conduits.

The veins of the human leg are better adapted to the erect posture than those of other mammals and it is often said that the calf muscle pump is a feature unique to man and his erect posture. This may not be entirely true as important features of the calf muscle pump, large venous sinsuses in the soleus and gastrocnemius muscles and the direct perforating veins, have been described in dissections of the hindleg of a quadrupedal macaque monkey (*Macaca fascicularis*)[1]. It can perhaps be argued that the human calf muscle pump is better developed than that of the macaque and that this development is in keeping with darwinian theory in being one of many factors which enabled primitive man to survive and dominate other species.

Blood is returned to the heart against gravity by a number of muscle pumps, most of which are illustrated in Figure 4.1. Three pumps which are not shown in this diagram are the foot pump, the abdominal pump and the respiratory pump. Gardner and Fox[2] have recently investigated the mechanism of the foot pump and have demonstrated that blood is expelled from the plantar veins by their intermittent stretching during foot movement, rather than by pressure of the sole of the foot on the ground. Their book, *The Return of Blood to the Heart*, also contains a chapter by Derek Griffiths which throws considerable doubt on the traditional concept of a respiratory pump. He argues that 'shallow inspiration probably does act to increase the total venous return slightly . . . but deep inspiration almost certainly reduces venous return'.

The capacity and pressure profiles of the calf muscle pump are outstandingly greater than all the other pumping mechanisms and its disordered function is the single most important factor in the aetiology of venous ulceration.

There are four important components of the calf muscle pump: the dilated valveless sinusoids within the soleus and gastrocnemius muscles, the direct perforating veins, the numerous valves in the communicating and deep veins which direct flow from superficial to deep and from distal to proximal, and the layer of

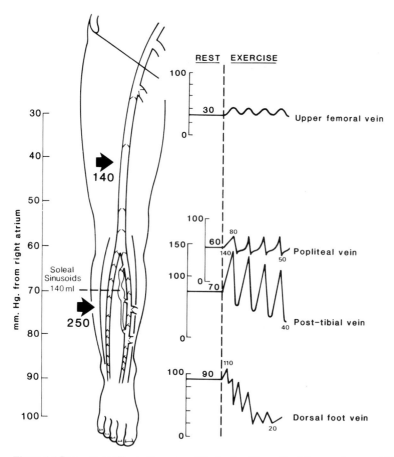

Figure 4.1 Pressure profiles in the veins of the foot, calf, popliteal fossa and upper thigh at rest and on walking. Foot venous pressure is progressively reduced by contractions of the calf muscle pump whose excursions of pressure are significantly greater than those of the popliteal or groin 'pumps'. The heavy black arrows indicate intramuscular pressures

very tough deep fascia which surrounds the calf muscles. This results in the high intramuscular pressures being transmitted directly to the soleal venous sinusoids.

The calf muscle pump has been described as a 'peripheral heart' and it may not be entirely coincidental that the total blood volume of the lower leg in the erect position is between 100 and 140 ml, very much the same as that of one of the ventricles. The calf muscles constitute a powerful pumping mechanism; intramuscular pressures of 250 mmHg have been measured by Ludbrook[3] and it is likely that venous pressures in the soleal sinusoids are similar, though these have not yet been directly measured. In the deep veins of the calf, which lie within the deep fascia but between the muscles, the pressures are rather less: Arnoldi has measured pressures of 140 mmHg in the posterior tibial veins of volunteers[4]. Pressure profiles at rest and during exercise in foot veins, the posterior tibial vein, the popliteal vein and the common femoral vein are shown in Figure 4.1. This is a composite diagram based on the work of Arnoldi and Ludbrook and on personal observations. The greatest pressure swings are seen in the posterior tibial vein. In the normal leg, the foot veins and tributaries of the calf and ankle perforating veins are protected by the integrity of their valves from the high systolic pressures produced by calf muscle contraction. During muscle relaxation (diastole), the valves prevent reflux and the calf muscle sinuses refill from the veins draining the calf muscles, from the foot veins and from the tributaries of the perforating veins on the medial and lateral surfaces of the ankle and lower leg. Note that, in the popliteal and femoral veins, resting pressures are significantly lower as the gravitational force is less here. The pressure exerted by the thigh muscles is also significantly less; unlike the calf muscles, these muscles are not completely enclosed in a rigid deep fascia. Although it has been suggested that all communicating veins, e.g. the long and short saphenous veins as well as the lower calf perforating veins, are subjected to high venous pressures in the presence of deep venous incompetence and reflux, this diagram illustrates that, when deep vein valves are incompetent, the pressures exerted on the lower calf and ankle perforating veins are significantly higher than those of either the long or short saphenous vein.

Calf muscle pump function is traditionally evaluated by foot venous pressure measurement in the erect posture (Figure 4.2); details of the method for measuring foot venous pressures are described in Chapter 7. Resting foot venous pressure reflects the height between the right atrium and foot and, in the erect position, is normally 80–90 mmHg. Following exercise, by raising the heel repeatedly off the ground, the pressure falls to about 25 mmHg (Figure 4.3). Standing motionless, the foot venous pressure takes 25–30 seconds to return to its previous high resting levels. Calf pump failure due to muscle weakness results in a poor exercising fall in

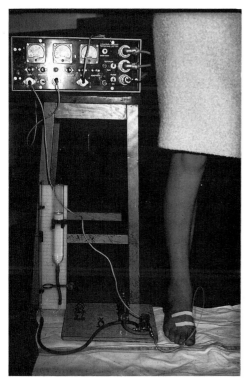

Figure 4.2 Foot venous pressure measurement. The pressure transducer is placed at foot level and after a stable resting pressure is achieved, foot venous pressure is reduced by repeated heel raising

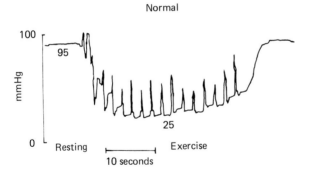

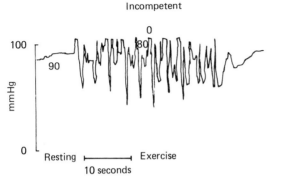

Figure 4.3 Normal and abnormal foot venous pressure profiles. In the lower trace, deep venous incompetence results in pressure swings with very little fall in mean pressure and a rapid return to high resting pressure

foot venous pressure; venous reflux results in a rapid return to resting pressure following exercise. There are now a number of non-invasive methods of measuring foot venous pressure and volume changes and these are also described in Chapter 7.

The disordered calf muscle pump

The calf muscle pump may become ineffective due to weakness of the muscles themselves, as may occur in paraplegia, multiple sclerosis or other neurological or muscular disorders. Alternatively, pump failure may result from venous obstruction or incompetence, most commonly the latter. The effects are markedly different. Patients with muscle weakness often develop oedema of the lower limb and ankle and this may be due as much to failure to pump tissue fluid along lymphatic trunks as to venous muscle pump inefficiency. Although some degree of oedema is usual, ulceration is extremely rare in these patients. Venous ulcers were called 'gravitational' by Dickson Wright[5] but, although paraplegic patients may develop leg ulcers, ambulatory venous hypertension is now considered the important factor in those with normal muscles but with peripheral venous incompetence.

The high venous pressures in the deep veins of the leg, which result from post-thrombotic recanalisation and valve incompetence, are unlikely to have any direct effect on the skin or subcutaneous tissues, from which they are separated by muscles and by a rigid deep fascia. There must be some pathway for conducting these high venous pressures to the subcutaneous tissues. In 1867 John Gay[6] questioned the relationship of ankle ulceration to varicose veins and described the ankle and calf perforating veins, and in 1917 John Homans[7] described the relationship of ankle ulceration to previous deep vein thrombosis. He divided leg ulcers into those associated with varicose veins, easily cured by removal of those veins, and post-phlebitic ulcers 'rapid in development, always intractable to palliative treatment, generally incurable by the removal of varicose veins alone, and must be excised to be cured'. It is worth noting that ulcer excision down to deep fascia will effectively excise the dilated veins which are the tributaries of the direct calf and ankle perforating veins and form the ankle flare. Turner Warwick[8] provided the first practical demonstration of flow from deep to superficial in incompetent perforating veins with his bleed back test and Cockett coined the descriptive term 'ankle blow-out' for direct perforating vein incompetence.

Over the years the emphasis has shifted from the gravitational pressure to ambulatory venous hypertension as a cause of venous ulceration. The enthusiasm which followed Linton and Cockett's operations for perforating vein ligation, and the disillusion which subsequently followed, have been described in Chapter 1 (page 6).

The case for the importance of direct perforating vein incompetence in the aetiology of venous ulceration is based on both theoretical considerations and clinical observations.

The role of perforating vein incompetence: theoretical considerations

Dodd and Cockett[9] made the important, and often overlooked, point that the direct perforating veins of the lower leg and ankle communicate with the main deep veins of the calf very close to their junction with the soleal arcades, which dilate to form the intramuscular soleal sinusoids (Figure 4.4). Incompetence of the perforating vein valves is therefore likely to transmit high exercising intramuscular pressures directly to their tributaries, the corona phlebectatica.

The measurement of dorsal foot venous pressures is often described as the gold standard of calf muscle pump function, although venous ulcers are extraordinarily rare on the dorsum of the foot. Most dorsal foot ulcers are ischaemic in origin. Most venous ulcers, on the other hand, are over the medial, or less commonly the lateral malleolus. These regions of the ankle are drained by a network of small tributaries of the direct perforating veins (the corona phlebectatica) which are not normally visible (see Figure 3.6). Following incompetence of the perforating vein, these venules dilate to become the ankle venous flare (Figure 4.5). This important physical sign is almost invariably seen before the development of lipodermatosclerosis or ulceration. Although these ankle venules communicate primarily with the deep veins through the direct perforating veins, they also communicate to a lesser degree with the long saphenous vein and, by way of the distal long saphenous vein, with the deep veins of the foot and leg through the metatarsal perforating veins (see Chapter 3).

Bjordal (1981)[10] performed direct measurements of pressure and flow in the superficial veins of the lower calf and ankle and demonstrated the transmission of

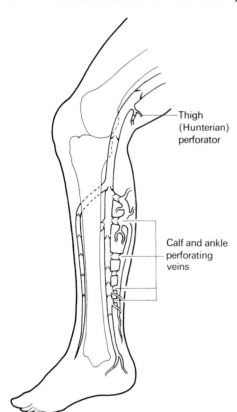

Thigh
(Hunterian)
perforator

Calf and ankle
perforating
veins

Figure 4.4 Diagram to demonstrate the close proximity of the direct perforating veins of the calf to the soleal sinusoids

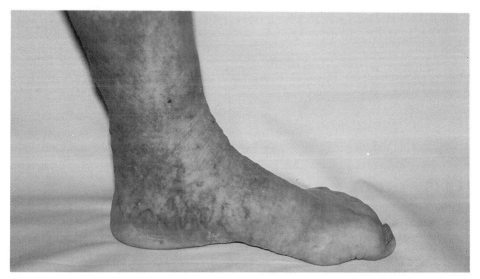

Figure 4.5 The ankle venous flare, an important physical sign indicating calf perforating vein incompetence

high pressures through incompetent perforating veins during muscle contraction, blood flow being inward during muscle relaxation and outward during contraction, with a nett outward flow of 60 ml/min. This would seem to be responsible for dilatation of the supramalleolar veins (the ankle venous flare), and these venules would seem to be mainly responsible for the microcirculatory changes which are responsible for lipodermatosclerosis and ulceration in the malleolar skin. The situation can be compared to a leaking bellows (Figure 4.6). The bellows with a damaged flap valve over its inlet hole will continue to eject air through its normal outlet, but air will also escape through the damaged inlet side hole. Substitute venous blood for air and the effect of perforating vein incompetence can be understood.

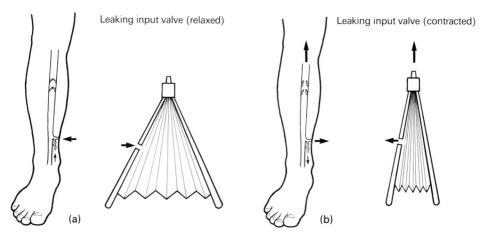

Figure 4.6 To illustrate the similarity between an incompetent direct calf perforating vein and a broken flap valve in a bellows: (a) in calf muscle relaxation, the reduced pressure in the deep veins 'sucks' blood from the superficial veins through the perforating veins (air is similarly 'sucked' into the bellows when it is expanded); (b) during muscle contraction, the perforating vein valve normally prevents blood refluxing to the superficial system but its incompetence allows reflux and the transmission of high pressures from the deep veins to the superficial (similarly air will escape through the broken side valve of the bellows as it is closed)

Clinical observations

Muscle weakness
Muscle weakness without venous damage may lead to oedema, but ulceration is rare.

Oedema of other causes
Ankle oedema resulting from renal or cardiac failure is only rarely accompanied by ulceration and ulcers are also rarely seen in lymphoedema.

Saphenous incompetence
Saphenous incompetence without perforating vein incompetence is very rarely associated with ulcer formation. Patients with very large and varicose tributaries of the saphenous systems for many years usually never develop ulceration. This is in

contrast to those with few, if any, varices but with an ankle venous flare denoting perforating vein incompetence, who almost invariably develop ulceration within a few years. In the Lewisham Hospital varicose vein clinic, the incidence of ulceration was observed in 113 patients with long saphenous incompetence of 153 legs and 24 ulcers were recorded. Calf or ankle perforating vein incompetence was detected in 19 of these 24 legs. Thus, only 5 ulcers (3.3%) were truly varicose in aetiology[11]. In a second series of 77 patients with 109 ulcerated legs, saphenous incompetence was found in only 36 (46.7%), all of whom had direct perforating vein incompetence[12].

Deep vein incompetence without perforating vein incompetence
This is an uncommon condition, as most patients with deep venous incompetence rapidly develop perforating vein incompetence, either because the thrombosis responsible for the deep venous incompetence also damages the perforating vein valves, or because the venous hypertension in the deep veins dilates the perforating veins so that their valves become secondarily incompetent. Patients with deep vein incompetence alone suffer from 'heaviness' of the legs on standing or walking, and often from calf swelling and ankle oedema. Liposclerosis or ulceration do not occur until perforating vein incompetence develops, and this can sometimes be delayed for many years by the use of compression stockings.

Perforating vein incompetence
The ankle venous flare is primarily the result of valve incompetence in the direct perforating veins of the lower calf and ankle (Figure 4.7a); the malleolar veins also communicate with the long saphenous vein, and therefore indirectly with the deep veins through the dorsal foot venous arch and metatarsal perforating veins. The incidence of direct perforating vein incompetence was studied by Doppler ultrasound and ascending venography in the author's series of 77 patients with 109 ulcerated legs. Perforating vein incompetence was diagnosed, and confirmed at operation, in 108 of the 109 legs. The exception was a patient who had previously undergone surgery to ligate incompetent perforating veins and whose ulceration was related to co-existent rheumatoid arthritis. Deep venous incompetence was found in less than half of these patients (32 patients; 44 legs)[12].

Deep venous obstruction
Patients with deep vein obstruction, most commonly due to failure of the left common iliac vein to recanalise (see Figure 3.12), suffer from swelling of the calf of the affected limb and also from 'bursting pain' on walking. The latter has been called venous claudication[13]. Proximal venous obstruction results in gradual distension of the peripheral deep and perforating veins and eventually in ulceration. This is common in patients with post-thrombotic iliac vein obstruction of ten or fifteen years' duration (see Figure 5.9), though ulceration is rarely seen in the first few years after iliofemoral thrombosis.

Perforating vein incompetence with deep venous incompetence and/or obstruction
This combination results in the most severe venous ulcers and the most resistant to treatment (Figure 4.7b, c). Burnand *et al.*[14] reported 100% ulcer recurrence within five years in a series of patients with phleobographic evidence of deep vein damage who were treated by direct perforating vein ligation. The same operation achieved very good results in other patients with venous ulcers in whom perforating vein

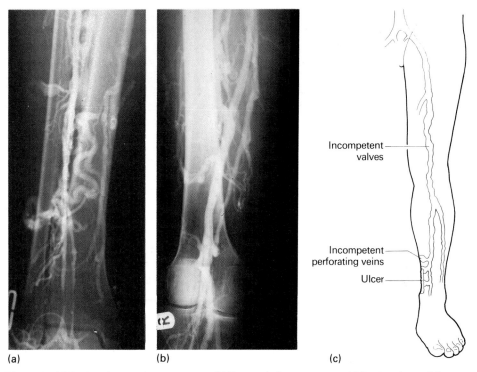

Figure 4.7 (a) Perforating vein incompetence. (b) Deep vein incompetence. (c) Perforating and deep vein incompetence

incompetence was accompanied by phlebographically normal deep veins. Neither group of patients wore elastic stockings post-operatively. It seems likely that the reason for ulcer recurrence following perforating vein ligation in the presence of deep venous incompetence and/or obstruction is that, in these patients, high venous pressure can still be transmitted to the ankle venous flare veins by the distal long saphenous vein through its communication with the plantar veins by way of the metatarsal communicating veins (see Chapter 3, page 17).

Improved results in patients with deep vein incompetence can be achieved by the addition of compression stockings following surgery, and these are described in detail in Chapter 10. It is unclear why knee-length compression stockings improve the results of perforating vein ligation. They may help by compressing the distal long saphenous vein on the foot and ankle, thus preventing high pressures in the deep veins from being transmitted to the ankle flare veins through the metatarsal perforating veins and the dorsal foot venous arch.

Summary

Calf muscle pump function may become disordered as a result of muscle weakness, saphenous incompetence, deep vein incompetence or obstruction, or perforating vein incompetence, with or without deep vein incompetence. All these abnormalities will adversely affect pressure profiles in the dorsal foot veins. Most venous ulcers occur in the malleolar regions which are drained by the corona phlebectatica, the network of small veins communicating with the calf and ankle perforating veins. In considering the pathophysiology of venous ulceration, as much attention must be paid to pressure and flow changes in this venous network, and to the factors influencing them, as to calf muscle pump function as evaluated by dorsal foot venous pressure measurement or alterations in foot volume.

At the present time, measurement of calf muscle pump function by dorsal foot venous pressure measurement or plethysmography, and its mathematical analysis, is not difficult. Measurement of flow and pressure changes in the ankle flare veins is extremely difficult, but it is likely that disorders in this venous network are of primary importance in the aetiology of venous ulceration. In the prevention of recurrent ulceration, all points of venous reflux communicating with the malleolar venous network must be accurately identified and effectively controlled.

References

1. Chappell, C. R., Wood, B. A. Venous drainage of the hind limb in the monkey. *J. Anat.* **131**: 157–171, 1980
2. Gardner, A. M. N., Fox, R. H. *The Return of Blood to the Heart,* London, Libbey, 1989
3. Ludbrook, J. *Aspects of Venous Function in the Lower Limbs,* Springfield, Illinois, Thomas, 1966
4. Arnoldi, C. C. Venous pressure in the leg of healthy human subjects at rest and during muscular exercise in the nearly erect position. *Acta Chir. Scand.* **130**: 570–583, 1965
5. Wright, A. D. Treatment of varicose ulcers. *Br. Med. J.* **2**: 996–998, 1930
6. Gay, J. On varicose disease of the lower extremities. *Lettsomian Lectures of 1867,* London, Churchill, 1868
7. Homans, J. The aetiology and treatment of varicose ulcers of the leg. *Surg. Gynecol. Obstet.* **24**: 300–311, 1917
8. Turner Warwick, W. *The Rational Treatment of Varicose Veins and Varicocele,* London, Faber, 1931
9. Dodd, H., Cockett, F. B. *The Pathology and Surgery of the Veins of the Lower Limb,* 2nd edn, Edinburgh, Churchill Livingstone, p. 38, 1976
10. Bjordal, R. I. Circulation patterns in incompetent perforating veins of the calf in venous dysfunction. In *Perforating Veins* (eds May, R., Partch, H., Staubesand, J), Munich, Urban and Schwarzenberg, p. 8, 1981
11. Negus, D. Perforating vein interruption in the post-phlebitic syndrome. In *Surgery of the Veins* (eds Bergen, J. J., Yao, J. S. T.), New York, Grune and Stratton, p. 195, 1985
12. Negus, D., Friedgood, A. The effective management of venous ulceration. *Br. J. Surg.* **70**: 623–625, 1983
13. Negus, D. Calf pain in the post-thrombotic syndrome. *Br. Med. J.* **2**: 156–158, 1968
14. Burnand, K. G., Thomas, M. L., O'Donnell, T., Brose, N. L. Relationship between post-phlebitic changes in the deep veins and results of surgical treatment of venous ulcers. *Lancet* **2**: 936–938, 1976

Chapter 5

The pathology of leg ulcers and of venous disorders

An ulcer has been defined as a 'discontinuity of an epithelial surface'[1]. A more descriptive definition is that of Sir Roy Cameron in Robbins' *Pathology*[2], 'an ulcer is a local defect, or excavation, of the surface of an organ or tissue, which is produced by the sloughing (shedding) of inflammatory necrotic tissue'.

The base of an ulcer consists of necrotic tissue and inflammatory exudate with variable degrees of fibroblastic proliferation and scarring. The surface always contains some bacteria and, in an acutely infected ulcer, these may proliferate to produce a purulent exudate. The base of a healing ulcer consists of bright red granulation tissue, the surface of the capillary loops arising from the dermal blood vessels (Figure 5.1).

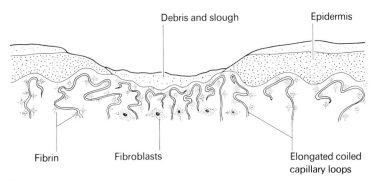

Figure 5.1 Diagrammatic cross-section of a healing venous ulcer

The edges are composed of epidermal cells attempting to migrate inwards to cover the granulation tissue and effect healing. Chronic ulceration occurs where epithelialisation of the edge and fibroblast proliferation in the base are opposed by factors preventing healing; in the leg these factors are usually vascular. Healing will be slow or non-existent when the arterial blood flow is insufficient to provide adequate metabolites for growth of the epithelial edge and the granulation tissue of the base; it will equally be deficient where venous hypertension opposes the process of tissue repair. Healing may also be inhibited by other factors such as infection, diabetes or the anti-inflammatory effect of steroid therapy; also vitamin C deficiency, anaemia and malnutrition.

Ischaemic ulceration

The base of an ischaemic ulcer has poorly formed, pale granulation tissue usually covered by necrotic slough (Figure 5.2). In the most severe, removal of this slough and debris will reveal the deep fascia or ankle tendons, with little or no granulation tissue. The edges are poorly epithelialised and there may be no visible epithelialisation at all, the base of the ulcer sharply demarcating into the surrounding ischaemic skin. Ischaemic ulceration is characterised by its site, in

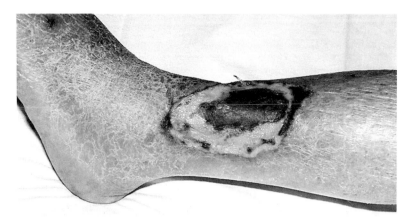

Figure 5.2 Ischaemic leg ulceration showing central gangrenous slough

areas of poor blood supply, and, where ulceration is secondary to major arterial disease, it is usually accompanied by ischaemic rest pain. Ischaemic ulceration most commonly results from atherosclerotic main vessel occlusion, but it can also arise from insufficiency of the small vessels, as in thromboangiitis obliterans (Buerger's disease), which is related to heavy cigarette smoking. Small vessel insufficiency also occurs in diabetic arteriopathy and vasculitis. Ulceration in patients suffering from these disorders, particularly diabetes, may result from a combination of large and small vessel disease. Care must be taken to detect peripheral pulses by palpation or by Doppler ultrasound in such patients, rather than dismissing them from consideration for arterial reconstructive surgery on the grounds that their arterial insufficiency is confined to small vessels and is therefore not suitable for surgical intervention. Care must also be taken to exclude arterial insufficiency in patients presenting with ulceration of predominantly venous origin. Concomitant arterial insufficiency is quite common in the elderly and attention must therefore be paid to treating both venous and arterial causes. Apparent foot ulceration may result from a sinus arising from underlying osteomyelitis and this possibility should always be checked by X-rays.

Venous ulcers

Venous ulcers most commonly occur over the medial malleolus and less frequently over the lateral surface of the ankle. A true varicose ulcer may lie anterior or posterior to these sites, usually directly over a large varix. However, anterior leg ulcers are much more likely to be ischaemic in origin and those on the dorsum of the foot are almost invariably ischaemic.

Venous ulcers vary in size from only a few centimetres (Figure 5.3) to giant ulcers which may be circumferential and involve the whole of the gaiter area of the lower leg (Figure 8.2). They are often infected when first seen but the infection responds rapidly to daily cleaning, non-irritant dressings, firm compression bandaging and appropriate antibiotics. This is in contrast to infected ischaemic ulcers, which

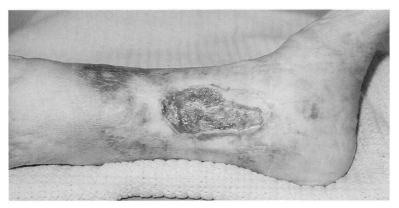

Figure 5.3 Venous ulcer

usually fail to respond to antibiotics until the ischaemia is successfully corrected. A clean venous ulcer has a base composed of healthy pink granulations covered perhaps by a little debris, and the edges consist of sloping pink epithelium. The granulation tissue represents the surface of capillary loops. A venous ulcer is usually surrounded by pigmented, indurated skin (lipodermatosclerosis), the result of peri-capillary fibrin deposition.

Bacteriology of leg ulcers

Most ulcers are infected when first seen. Opinions differ about whether such infection is primary or secondary, but it seems likely that infection is usually secondary to the underlying venous or arterial disorder. Minor skin abrasions are invariably accompanied by the entry of a few skin bacteria whose colonisation can proceed unimpeded in the presence of ischaemia or venous hypertension.

The organisms cultured are mostly Gram-positive skin organisms. A random survey of the bacteriological findings in 30 leg ulcers in patients attending clinics at Lewisham Hospital between May and September 1989 is shown in Table 5.1. *Staphylococcus aureus* is the most commonly cultured organism. Coliforms were never cultured alone, but were always found in combination with a Gram-positive organism, usually *Staph. aureus*. Coliforms were occasionally found with other organisms, streptococcus in three cultures and *Staph. albus* in one. Anaerobic organisms were not looked for in these bacteriological examinations, but Browse and his colleagues[3] did investigate their presence and found them in 44% of the ulcers cultured. For this reason, it is always wise to prescribe metronidazole in addition to antibiotics specific for aerobic organisms.

Table 5.1 Bacteriological findings in 30 leg ulcers

Organism cultured	No. of cases
Single	
Staph. aureus	9
Pseudomonas aeruginosa	4
Strep. faecalis	1
Diphtheroids (+ Staph. albus)	1
Coliforms (+ Staph. albus)	1
Multiple	
Staph. aureus + coliform	5
Staph. aureus + diphtheroids	1
Staph. aureus + Strep. faecalis	1
Staph. aureus + β-haemolytic strep.	1
Staph. aureus + β-haemolytic strep. + pseudomonas	1
Staph. aureus + E. coli + group B strep.	1
β-Haemolytic strep. + P. aeruginosa	1
β-Haemolytic strep. + P. aeruginosa + coliform	1
Strep. faecalis + coliform	1
Strep. viridans + coliform + diphtheroids	1

Venous disorders responsible for ulceration

Although varicose eczema is a common complication of varicose veins, true varicose ulcers are rare and were described by Homans in 1916[4] as being superficial and easily cured by removal of the varicose veins, in contrast to post-phlebitic ulcers. Many patients with large dilated varicose veins (Figure 5.4) never develop ulceration, even after many years. Our own findings in 113 patients with long saphenous incompetence of 153 legs have been described in Chapter 4. Only 24 legs were ulcerated and perforating vein incompetence was detected in 19 of these.

Although true varicose ulcers are uncommon, varicose veins may be responsible for venous ulceration in the malleolar skin by their effect in dilating the valve rings of calf and ankle perforating veins and rendering these incompetent. It is therefore appropriate to discuss the pathological changes which result in varicose dilatation.

Varicose veins

Varicose veins are defined as distended, elongated, tortuous superficial veins with incompetent valves. It has been supposed that valvular incompetence starts at the saphenofemoral junction and may be the result of pressure from a gravid uterus or even from pressure produced by the constipated sigmoid colon. The statement that 'varicose veins are the penalty that man pays for assuming the upright posture' forgets that there are many mammals with longer legs and therefore potentially greater foot venous pressures than man.

Rare among rural Africans and Indians, primary familial varicose veins are very common indeed in industrialised Western society. A number of studies from Europe and North and South America have described an incidence of about 50% in the middle-aged and elderly with about a 10% greater incidence in women[5]. It is

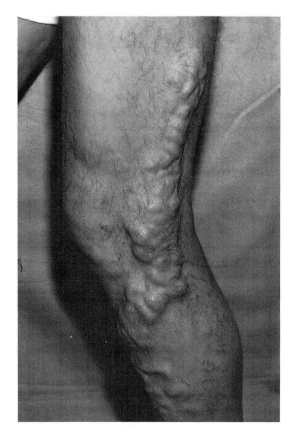

Figure 5.4 Gross varicose veins of the long saphenous system

unlikely that primary varicose veins occur as the result of valve defects, as varicose blow-outs can quite often be found distal to intact valves[6]. Tensiometer studies have demonstrated that the valve is the single strongest part of the vein[7]. High venous pressure resulting from primary valve failure also seems less likely as a cause of varicosity when it is remembered that the saphenous vein used as an arterial conduit becomes thick walled and arterialised, rather than thin walled and varicose.

Histological observations
In 1963 Svejcar *et al.*[8] described deficient collagen in the walls of varicose veins and also showed that the same defect was present in undilated veins and in the arm veins of the same subject. Histological studies by Haardt[9] and Rose[6] have also demonstrated that the smooth muscle coats are disorganised; normal longitudinal and circular muscle fibres can no longer be distinguished and areas of muscle are broken up by disorganised collagen (Figure 5.5). This disorganisation of vein wall architecture would seem to be responsible for the decrease in elasticity observed in the walls of varicose veins[10].

Catabolism of connective tissue in patients with primary varicose veins is greater than in normal controls[11]. This is associated with increased lysosomal activity[12] and to an increase in serum levels of these enzymes[13]. Haardt[9], in addition to

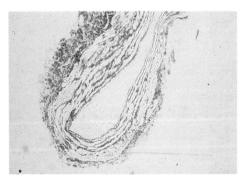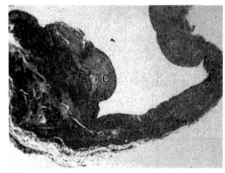

Figure 5.5 (a) Normal vein: layers of smooth muscle are separated by well-organised bands of collagen and elastic tissue (Elastic van Gieson; ×10). (b) Varicose vein showing grossly disorganised collagen and fragmented areas of smooth muscle, with an abnormal subintimal collagen deposit (H & E; × 10)

demonstrating the histological features of varicose veins, has also undertaken elegant histochemical studies in which he has demonstrated not only an increase in the collagen-splitting enzymes in the connective tissue of the vein wall, but also a decrease in phosphatases in the muscle coats. He suggests that the weakness of varicose vein walls is the result not only of anatomical disorganisation of structure, but also of muscle weakness due to lack of energy-producing enzymes involved in the Krebs' cycle.

Patients with primary varicose veins usually have a strong family history of the problem (usually in the mother), and these observations seem to provide a more acceptable hypothesis for the aetiology of varicose veins than dubious explanations based on 'the penalty for assuming the upright posture', 'constipation', or 'pressure of the gravid uterus'. However, they fail to explain varicose veins secondary to deep vein thrombosis or arteriovenous fistula formation, or why the long and short saphenous systems may become varicose independently of each other.

Varicose veins in pregnancy
Varicose veins are more commmon in women than in men and usually appear for the first time during the first pregnancy. They often disappear after the baby is born, only to reappear and persist during and after the second pregnancy. Pressure of the gravid uterus seems unlikely to be responsible as varicose veins usually appear relatively early during pregnancy and it is unlikely that the uterus exerts any significant pressure on the pelvic veins until the head engages in the pelvis shortly before parturition.

A more plausible explanation is that the veins, with their already weakened walls, become further weakened and dilated in response to increased oestrogen and progesterone levels, which are recognised to cause smooth muscle and collagen weakness, resulting in ureteric dilatation and softening of the pelvic ligaments. Pregnancy is accompanied by an increase in plasma volume, which reaches a maximum of 49% of the non-pregnant plasma volume shortly before parturition[14]. Two-thirds of the circulating blood volume is contained in the veins, the capacitance vessels. The combination of vein wall weakness and an increase in the contained volume would seem to be responsible for the varicose dilatation, which often persists after pregnancy, particularly after the second pregnancy.

Varieties of varicose veins

Varicose veins may present as small local varices without evidence of either long or short venous incompetence. Much more common are those associated with long stem incompetence and reflux. The long saphenous vein itself is only rarely dilated and incompetent in the lower leg. Most calf varices are dilated tributaries which join the long saphenous vein at knee level. Ankle varices may be related to calf perforating vein incompetence, but incompetent perforating veins are often without varicose tributaries; they are more frequently demonstrated only by a malleolar venous flare.

The post-thrombotic syndrome and perforating vein incompetence

Following thrombosis, fibroblasts, mast cells, polymorphs and histiocytes invade the vein wall and the occluded lumen is usually restored by a combination of thrombus retraction and recanalisation (Figure 5.6). Post-thrombotic deep venous incompetence, often accompanied by perforating vein incompetence and sometimes by secondary varices, results from pathological changes of the vein wall entirely different to those of varicose veins. Instead of the vein wall becoming thin

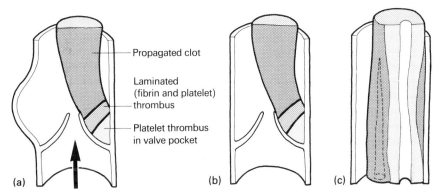

Figure 5.6 The natural history of venous thrombosis. (a) Thrombus formation in a valve pocket; the lines of Zahn (fibrin) are separated by platelet accumulations and these together form the 'white head', which is followed by the tail of propagated clot. (b) Organisation; infiltration by histiocytes, mast cells and fibroblasts. (c) Post-thrombotic thrombus retraction and recanalisation, resulting in valve incompetence

and weak, as in primary varicose veins, the walls of previously thrombosed veins are thicker and less distensible than those of normal veins, due to collagen deposition by fibroblasts in the process of recanalisation. The lumen is usually patent but irregular. In the process of recanalisation, the delicate valves are either destroyed or become permanently adherent to the adjacent vein wall (Figure 5.7). Venous incompetence is therefore the direct result of valve incompetence, rather than vein wall dilatation resulting in incompetence of normal valves, as in varicose veins.

Homans[4] description of the post-phlebitic syndrome was an important step in directing attention away from the concept of varicose ulceration but it has subsequently become clear that by no means all patients with venous ulceration have a past history of deep vein thrombosis. In 1942 Bauer[15] found that 87% of 38

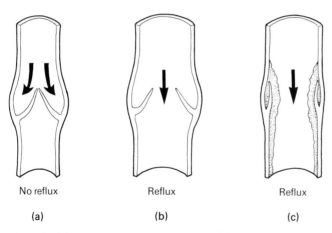

No reflux   Reflux   Reflux

(a)   (b)   (c)

Figure 5.7 (a) Normal venous valve, no reflux. (b) Dilated varicose vein, normal valve cusps but fail to meet, reflux. (c) Post-thrombotic recanalisation with adherent valve cusps, reflux

patients with venous ulcers gave a definite history of previous thrombosis, but Dodd, in 1954 (cited in Dodd and Cockett[16]), found such a history in only 30% of 121 cases of venous ulceration.

In the Lewisham Hospital series of 77 patients with venous ulcers, a past history of venous thrombosis was found in 45 (58%)[17]. Although previous deep vein thrombosis has been discounted as an inevitable cause of venous ulceration, perforating vein incompetence is usually found in such cases. In 1953, Cockett[18] explored the perforating veins of 135 limbs with lipodermatosclerosis and ulceration and, using the Turner Warwick bleed back test, found 96 of these to be incompetent. The incidence of saphenous and perforating vein incompetence was investigated in the Lewisham Hospital series of 77 patients[17]; incompetent direct calf and ankle perforating veins were demonstrated by Doppler ultrasound and confirmed at operation in 108 of 109 ulcerated legs. In this series, deep venous incompetence was diagnosed in only 32 (42%).

Direct perforating vein incompetence may arise from one of the following causes, or from a combination of these.

1. Long-standing primary varicose veins with long or short saphenous incompetence; the varicose perforating vein dilates and its valve becomes incompetent in the same way as in other primary varicose veins.
2. Following local thrombophlebitis, with racanalisation and valve damage, which in turn usually follows local trauma.
3. Following deep vein thrombosis and recanalisation. The perforating veins are very often involved in such thrombosis and recanalisation and their valves are damaged in this process. Alternatively, even if the individual perforating vein is not thrombosed, incompetence of and reflux down the deep veins with which it communicates may lead to dilatation of its valve ring and therefore to secondary incompetence. Ulcers resulting from the combined effects of perforating vein and deep vein incompetence are the most difficult to treat and the most likely to recur[19].

Post-thrombotic venous occlusion

Post-thrombotic recanalisation occasionally fails, leaving permanent venous stenosis or occlusion. This most commonly affects the left common iliac vein (Figure 5.8) and this is related to the anatomical anomalies which are described in Chapter 3. Venous occlusion occasionally occurs elsewhere, particularly in the superficial femoral vein. Main vessel occlusion is often adequately compensated by

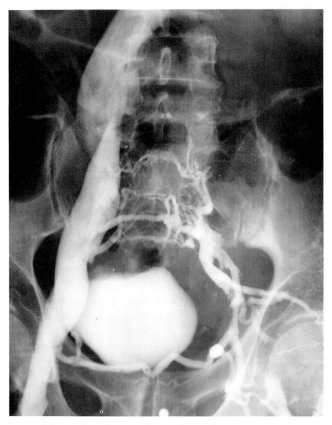

Figure 5.8 Post-thrombotic occlusion of the left common and external iliac veins; collateral flow through pudendal and presacral tributaries of the internal iliac veins

the development of numerous collateral veins, but failure of adequate collateral vein development results in functional obstruction to the venous return. Venography will show the site of venous occlusion, but cannot indicate its functional significance, and physiological investigations by femoral venous pressure measurements[20], plethysmography or Duplex scanning are required for full evaluation.

The high exercising venous pressure which follows proximal venous obstruction causes distension of the deep veins. Intramuscular pressure in the calf muscles is elevated during exercise in legs with outflow obstruction[21] and muscle water content is also increased, probably due to increased transudation of fluid[22]. An increased interstitial pressure may lead to compression of the distal end of the capillaries resulting in the increased fluid transudation and increase in muscle water content. Capillary compression would also seem the reason for the reduced exercising muscle blood flow and increase in lactate content in the gastrocnemius muscles of legs with iliac occlusion and outflow obstruction[21]. These changes are responsible for pain on exercise (venous claudication).

Patients with post-thrombotic iliac vein obstruction rarely develop ulceration in the first five years following thrombosis. Ulceration becomes much more common after ten or fifteen years (Figure 5.9) and results from the development of secondary incompetence of the peripheral deep and perforating veins and often also of the saphenous veins.

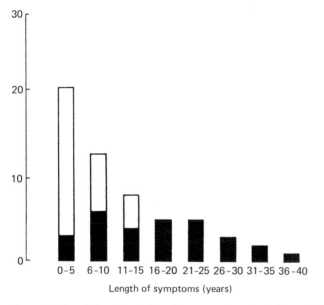

Figure 5.9 The relationship of ulceration to post-thrombotic iliac occlusion. □, Total patients in each group; ■, number of patients with ulcers

Important collaterals in common iliac occlusion have been described in Chapter 3. In the thigh, the collateral pathways which usually compensate for occlusion of the superficial femoral vein are the profunda femoris vein and the long saphenous vein. Care must be taken not to ligate the latter in patients with post-thrombotic stenosis or occlusion of the superficial femoral vein.

The microcirculation in venous ulceration

Although there is little doubt that venous ulceration results from high ambulatory venous pressures in the subcutaneous veins of the lower leg and ankle, there is still controversy about the precise effect of such pressure on the skin microcirculation. The three current theories are the fibrin cuff theory, white cell entrapment and microthrombus formation.

Fibrin cuff theory

Histological examination of the subepidermal capillary bed in patients with venous hypertension was initially thought to show an increased number of capillaries[23], but subsequent observations have suggested that the rise in venous pressure causes dilatation of the horizontal subcapillary venous plexus[24, 25] with grossly coiled, elongated capillary loops and a reduction in the number of capillaries supplying the epidermis. Burnand et al.[26], showed that fibrinogen 'leaks' from these dilated capillaries, forming a pericapillary fibrin cuff, which was thought to be responsible for reduced diffusion of blood oxygen to tissues. This subcutaneous fibrin deposition results in induration, with brown pigmentation (haemosiderin), which often precedes or surrounds a venous ulcer. Originally termed 'fat necrosis', the fibrin cuff hypothesis has given birth to the new name, lipodermatosclerosis; liposclerosis for short. In its acute inflammatory form, it can be very painful and tender. Both systemic and tissue fibrinolytic activity is significantly reduced in patients with venous hypertension[27].

The hypothesis that the fibrin cuff forms a diffusion barrier to oxygen is supported by Blalock's observation[28] that the venous blood leaving an ulcerated limb has a high oxygen content; it is also supported by skin blood flow measurements and measurements of oxygen utilization in patients with lipo-dermatosclerosis and ulceration, using positron emission tomography[29]. This method has demonstrated reduced tissue extraction of oxygen in cases of lipodermatosclerosis and in the skin at the edge of ulcers. Recently, Mani and his colleagues[30] found skin oxygen tension at ulcer edges to be significantly lower than that of control (apparently normal) skin in legs with venous incompetence. However, skin oxygen tension in the latter is lower than that in healthy volunteers. This suggests that factors other than fibrin cuff (perhaps oedema) may also reduce oxygen tension. The problem is further complicated by the poor arteriolar supply of the skin in the ulcer-bearing area of the leg[31].

The hypothesis that fibrin cuff formation, by preventing oxygen and metabolite transfer to the overlying skin, is responsible for lipodermatosclerosis and subsequent ulceration, is attractive and brings together a number of previously unexplained observations. It may not be the whole story, as lipodermatosclerosis is by no means invariably followed by ulceration and venous ulcers are not always surrounded by obviously liposclerotic skin.

White cell entrapment

An alternative hypothesis has recently been suggested by Coleridge Smith and his colleagues[32]. Bollinger et al.[33], using capillary fluorescence microscopy in patients with chronic venous insufficiency, observed areas of ankle skin with no apparent blood flow. Using the same technique, Scott et al.[34] found that the number of functioning capillary loops visible in the skin fell after the legs had been dependent for thirty minutes. It has also been demonstrated[35] that leucocytes become trapped in the circulation of dependent legs. It has therefore been suggested that, by linking these two findings, trapped white cells occlude capillaries, resulting in localised areas of ischaemia, which in turn lead to ulceration.

Scott and his colleagues[36] have observed that changes in posture do not cause a significant fluctuation in the systemic haematocrit or white cell:red cell ratio. They found this to be true in both their control group of patients and also in those with chronic venous insufficiency and they conclude that 'this is fortunate since if the large numbers of white cells that Thomas et al.[35] found to be trapped were lost in every part of the lower limb circulation (30% of the entering white blood cells), the systemic blood would rapidly become depleted of white blood cells. Clearly white cell trapping occurs on only a small part of the lower limb, perhaps just that area of skin immediately proximal to the malleoli. We were unable to show white cell trapping in blood taken from the foot, even in patients with chronic venous insufficiency'. These observations provide tentative support for the hypothesis that the ankle venous flare, resulting from high ambulatory venous pressures transmitted through incompetent perforating veins, is the venous bed most affected by ambulatory venous hypertension and this results in lipodermatosclerosis and ulceration affecting overlying malleolar skin. Unfortunately, Scott and his colleagues found cannulation of the long saphenous vein in the gaiter region impossible due to thickened, hard lipodermatosclerotic skin. The hypothesis that white cell entrapment may be responsible for the disappearance of capillary loops and may contribute to liposclerosis and ulceration depends on demonstrating that white cells are actually trapped in the malleolar venous flare veins. Hopefully, future attempts at sampling will be more successful.

Microthrombosis

It has been suggested by Ehrly and Partsch[37] that impaired perfusion, leading to tissue hypoxia, may be in part due to the development of microthrombi in the underlying vascular bed. Ehrly and colleagues have suggested that long-term stimulation of fibrinolysis by low-dose urokinase can increase $TcPo_2$ values and lead to a reduction in ulcer area[38].

All three mechanisms, and perhaps others, may be responsible for skin hypoxia and ulceration. Whatever the precise mechanism, the message is clear: all these hypotheses depend on the common denominator of venous hypertension and any approach to healing venous ulcers must aim to counteract such venous hypertension. In the healing stage of management, this hypertension is counteracted by appropriate elastic compression bandages or stockings; in definitive treatment and in the prevention of recurrent ulceration, attention must be paid to identifying all points of venous incompetence responsible for such hypertension and correcting these by appropriate measures in each case.

References

1. Harding Rains, A. J., Mann, C. V. (eds) *Bailey and Love's Short Practice of Surgery,* London, Lewis, p. 113, 1988
2. Robbins, S. L. *Pathology,* Philadelphia, Saunders, p. 58, 1967
3. Browse, N. L., Burnand, K. G., Lea Thomas, M. *Diseases of the Veins; Pathology, Diagnosis and Treatment,* London, Arnold, p. 406, 1988
4. Homans, J. The operative treatment of varicose veins and ulcers, based on a classification of these lesions. *Surg. Gynecol. Obstet.* **22**: 143–158, 1916
5. Franks, P. J., Wright, D. D. I., McCollum, C. N. Epidemiology of venous disease: a review. *Phlebology,* **4**: 143–151, 1989
6. Rose, S. S. The aetiology of varicose veins. In *Phlebology '85* (eds Negus, D., Jantet, G.), London, Libbey, pp. 6–9, 1986

7. Ackroyd, J. S., Patterson, M., Browse, N. L. A study of the mechanical properties of fresh and preserved human femoral vein wall and valve cusps. *Br. J. Surg.* **72**: 117–119, 1985
8. Svejcar, J., Prerovsky, I., Linhart, J., *et al.* Content of collagen, elastin and hexosamine in primary varicose veins. *Clin. Sci.* **24**: 325–330, 1963
9. Haardt, B. A comparison of the histochemical enzyme pattern in normal and varicose veins. *Phlebology* **2**: 135–158, 1987
10. Thulesius, O., Gjöres, J. E., Berlin, E. Valvular function and venous distensibility. *Phlebology '85* (eds Negus, D., Jantet, G.), London, Libbey, pp. 26–28, 1986
11. Buddecke, E. Alters Veränderungen der Proteoglykane verh deutsch. *Ges. Pathol.* **59**: 43, 1975
12. Niebes, P., Laszt, L. Influence in-vitro d'une série de flavinoides sur des enzymes du métabolisme des mucopolysaccharides de veines saphènes humaines et bovines. *Angiologia* **8**: 297–302, 1971
13. Niebes, P., Berson, I. *Determination of Enzymes and Degradation.* London, Churchill Livingstone, p. 35, 1976
14. Documenta Geigy. *Scientific Tables* (ed. Diem, K.), Macclesfield, Geigy, p. 604, 1962
15. Bauer, G. A roentgenological and clinical study of the sequels of thrombosis. *Acta Chir. Scand.* **86**: Suppl. 74, 1942
16. Dodd, H., Cockett, F. B. *The Pathology and Surgery of the Veins of the Lower Limb,* 2nd edn, Edinburgh, Churchill Livingstone, p. 247, 1976
17. Negus, D., Friedgood, A. The effective management of venous ulceration. *Br. J. Surg.* **70**: 623–625, 1983
18. Cockett, F. B. Pathology and treatment of venous ulcers. *Thesis*, University of London, 1953
19. Burnand, K. G., Lea Thomas, M., O'Donnell, P., Browse, N. L. Relationship between post-phlebitic changes in the deep veins and results of surgical treatment of venous ulcers. *Lancet* **2**: 936–938, 1976
20. Negus, D., Cockett, F. B. Femoral vein pressures in post-phlebitic iliac vein obstruction. *Br. J. Surg.* **54**: 522–525, 1967
21. Qvarfordt, P., Eklöf, B., Ohlin, P., Plate, G., Saltin, B. Intramuscular pressure, blood flow and skeletal muscle metabolism in patients with venous claudication. *Surgery* **95**: 191–195, 1984
22. Zelis, R., Lee, G., Mason, D. T. Influence of experimental edema on metabolically determined blood flow. *Circ. Res.* **34**: 482–489, 1974
23. Whimster, I. Quoted in *The Pathology and Surgery of the Veins of the Lower Limb,* 2nd edn (eds Dodd, H., Cockett, F. B.), Edinburgh, Churchill Livingstone, p. 258, 1976
24. Fagrell, B. Vital capillary microscopy. *Scand. J. Clin. Lab. Invest.* suppl. 133, 2–50, 1973
25. Ryan, T. J. The epidermis and its blood supply in venous disorders of the leg. *Trans. St. John's Hosp. Dermatol. Soc.* **55**: 51–63, 1969
26. Burnand, K. G., Whimster, I., Naidoo, A., Browse, N. L. Pericapillary fibrin in the ulcer-bearing skin of the leg: the cause of lipodermatosclerosis and venous ulceration. *Br. Med. J.* **285**: 1071–1072, 1982
27. Layer, G. T., Pattison, M., Evans, B. *et al.* Varicose veins. In *Phlebology '85* (eds Negus, D., Jantet, G.), London, Libbey, pp. 10–12, 1986
28. Blalock, A. Oxygen content of blood in patients with varicose veins. *Arch. Surg.* **19**: 898–905, 1929
29. Hopkins, N. F. G., Spinks, T. J., Rhodes, C. G., Ranicar, A. S. O., Jamieson, C. W. Positron emission tomography in venous ulceration and liposclerosis, a study of regional tissue function. *Br. Med. J.* **286**: 323–336, 1983
30. Mani, R., White, J. E., Barratt, D. F., Weaver, P. W. Tissue oxygenation, venous ulcers and fibrin cuffs. *J. R. Soc. Med.* **82**: 345–346, 1989
31. Edwards, D. A. W. Quoted in *The Pathology and Surgery of the Veins of the Lower Limb,* 2nd edn (eds Dodd, H. and Cockett, F. B.), Edinburgh, Churchill Livingstone, p. 49, 1976
32. Coleridge Smith, P. D., Thomas, P., Scurr, J. H., Dormandy, J. A. Causes of venous ulceration; a new hypothesis. *Br. Med. J.* **296**: 1726–1727, 1988
33. Bollinger, A., Haselbach, D., Schnewling, G., Jünger, M. Microangiopathy due to chronic venous incompetence evaluated by fluorescence videomicrosocpy. In *Phlebology '85* (eds Negus, D., Jantet, G.), London, Libbey, pp. 751–753, 1986
34. Scott, H. J., McMullin, G.M., Coleridge Smith, P. D., Scurr, J. H. The microcirculation and

venous ulceration in the skin of the calf. In *Phlébologie '89* (eds Davy, A., Stemmer, R.), Paris, Libbey, pp. 282–284, 1989

35. Thomas, P. R. S., Nash, G. B., Dormandy, J. A. White cell accumulation in dependent legs of patients with venous hypertension: a possible mechanism for trophic changes in the skin. *Br. Med. J.* **296**: 1693–1695, 1988

36. Scott, H. J., McMullin, G. M., Coleridge Smith, P. D., Scurr, J. H. Venous ulceration: the role of the white blood cell. *Phlebology* **4**: 153–159, 1989

37. Ehrly, A. M., Partsch, H. Microcirculatory and haemorrheological abnormalities in venous leg ulcers: introductory remarks. In *Phlébologie '89* (eds Davy, A., Stemmer, R.), Paris, Libbey, pp. 142–145, 1989

38. Ehrly, A. M., Schenk, J., Bromberger, W. The effects of low dose, long term urokinase on TcPo$_2$ of patients with venous leg ulcers. In *Phlébologie '89* (eds Davy, A., Stemmer, R.), Paris, Libbey, pp. 147–149, 1989

Part II

Practical applications

Chapter 6

Diagnosis: history and examination

Energetic attempts to heal ulcers and to prevent their recurrence are often unsuccessful due to the failure to appreciate that diagnosis and treatment of the underlying cause of the ulcer is very much more important than treatment of the ulcer itself. Even when this concept has been grasped, accurate diagnosis may be hampered by lack of familiarity with methods of investigation. The most frequent error is the failure to recognise that an ulcer is ischaemic in origin, and many ischaemic ulcers are undoubtedly made much worse by tight compression bandaging, in the mistaken belief that they are venous. As the latter are by far the most common, this is an understandable mistake, but in an ageing and cigarette-smoking society, ischaemic ulceration is now seen with increasing frequency.

History

In taking the patient's history it is important to note the duration of the ulcer, whether there was any precipitating cause, and whether there is any past history of deep vein thrombosis or varicose veins. It is also important to enquire whether the patient has experienced symptoms suggestive of ischaemia, intermittent claudication or rest pain. A venous ulcer may be locally painful, but if the patient complains of pain in the toes or forefoot, suspect ischaemia. Remember that the history may sometimes be misleading; a history of deep vein thrombosis does not necessarily mean that the ulcer is venous in origin. A typical example is that of a 54-year-old man whose ulcer had been treated for some years by compression bandaging because he had suffered a deep vein thrombosis in the distant past. Examination showed absolutely no evidence of deep vein disorder, ankle pulses were absent, and the ulcer was obviously ischaemic. Ulcers of mixed venous and arterial origin are not uncommon, particularly in the elderly, and a history of deep vein thrombosis or varicose veins may co-exist with symptoms of intermittent claudication and ischaemic rest pain. Even the symptom of pain on walking, claudication, may cause diagnostic confusion as post-thrombotic venous obstruction may result in severe calf pain on walking, so-called venous claudication[1].

Where the history, examination and investigations show no evidence of either venous or arterial cause, other possibilities must be considered. These include rheumatoid arthritis and the hands and other joints should be examined for evidence of arthritis in all ulcer patients. Diabetic ulcers are usually on the sole of the foot, but may occur on the leg, and all new patients attending an ulcer clinic must have a routine urine check. Other forms of vasculitis may sometimes present with leg ulcers and these are considered in more detail in Chapter 8. Suspect vitamin C deficiency in the elderly who live alone and whose diet may be inadequate. The possibility of an ulcer being malignant must always be borne in mind and a biopsy performed if there is any doubt. Hypertension may occasionally present with leg ulceration, though there is some doubt whether the ulcer described by Martorell is in fact a distinct entity. Patients may not volunteer a history of hypertension, but careful questioning will usually discover whether they are taking diuretics or anti-hypertensive drugs.

Examination

A full general examination must be carried out and this must include blood pressure measurement and urine testing. Examine the conjunctivae for evidence of anaemia. Leg pulses must be palpated in all patients, in order to avoid overlooking this important step in the elderly, whose ulcers are more likely to be ischaemic in origin. Ankle pulses are often difficult to feel in the ulcerated and oedematous leg and Doppler ultrasound examination must then be used.

Careful abdominal examination must be performed to exclude abdominal aortic aneurysm or other abdominal masses. Rectal examination should also be performed, particularly in any patient presenting with a swollen leg. Some textbook accounts still attribute primary varicose veins to compression of venous return by an abdominal tumour. It seems more likely that primary familial varicose veins are the result of an inherited collagen and smooth muscle defect in the vein wall (see Chapter 5) and any abdominal mass in such patients is likely to be coincidental. However leg swelling can certainly occur as a result of iliac vein compression by tumour spread, particularly if this involves perivenous lymph nodes. Carcinoma of the prostate must therefore be excluded in men and uterine or ovarian malignancy in women.

During abdominal examination, the groins must be carefully examined for the presence of dilated collateral veins, the result of iliac venous occlusion. These most often appear as dilated subcutaneous veins rather than true varices. If they are present, or if the patient's history suggests an episode of iliofemoral deep vein thrombosis, calf circumference should be measured to see whether there is any discrepancy. Post-thrombotic iliac vein occlusion, and its attendant physical signs, most often affects the left leg (Figure 6.1).

The colour and temperature of the toes gives a good indication of blood flow. Both patients with venous insufficiency and those with ischaemia may have cyanosed feet, but cyanosis secondary to venous congestion will show rapid refilling after firm finger pressure to empty the superficial vessels, while an ischaemic foot will have a slow refilling time, as long as 4 or 5 seconds. Following abdominal and pedal pulse examination, careful attention should be paid to the site and appearance of the ulcer itself. These features are dealt with in detail in Chapter 8. It can however be broadly stated that venous ulcers most commonly occur in the skin over the malleoli, most usually the medial, and often occur in an area of lipodermatosclerosis or pigmentation. Ischaemic ulcers are usually on the anterior surface of the leg and dorsum of the foot and diabetic ulcers are most commonly on the sole of the foot. Ulcers are however notorious mimics and it is quite common

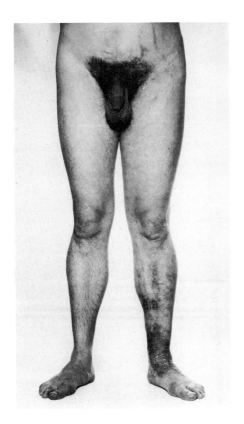

Figure 6.1 Dilated groin collaterals and a swollen leg secondary to post-thrombotic iliac vein occlusion

for an ischaemic ulcer to occur over the medial malleolus, to all appearances looking exactly like a venous ulcer. A typical example was a young Arab soldier with a two-year history of ankle ulceration. He had a history of deep vein thrombosis following a comminuted fracture of the left ankle. Examination showed a typical venous ulcer over the medial malleolus and he was treated for several months by bed rest, elevation, dressings and compression bandages. The ulcer failed to heal and he was then referred to the author's clinic. The posterior tibial pulse could not be felt and was therefore checked by Doppler ultrasound examination. This also failed to detect a pulse and subsequent arteriography showed occlusion of the posterior tibial artery, a previously overlooked complication of his fracture. Doppler ultrasound also demonstrated perforating vein incompetence. The ulcer healed following ligation of the incompetent perforating vein and chemical lumbar sympathectomy to improve arterial blood flow to the ankle.

Following general and pedal pulse examination on the examination couch, the patient is asked to stand so that thorough examination of the leg veins can be performed. An 18 cm (7 in) high mounting block is essential to avoid backache in the examiner, and even elderly patients are able to stand on such a low platform with adequate support (Figure 6.2). A good standard lamp is also essential. Those who design out-patient clinics seem to assume that all examinations are performed with the patient on the couch and usually only provide a wall lamp.

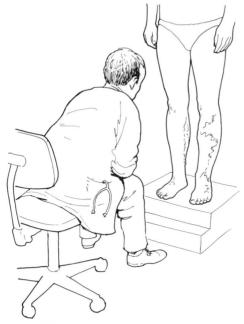

Figure 6.2 Examination. A suitable platform and good light are essential

The lower leg and foot are first inspected for evidence of cyanosis, which may not have been evident in the supine position, particularly if venous in origin. The surroundings of the ulcer are carefully inspected for evidence of lipodermatoscler-osis or pigmentation, typical of the venous ulcer, and the malleolar skin is equally carefully inspected for the presence or absence of an ankle venous flare (Figure 6.3). This fine network of venules, which has been described as the corona

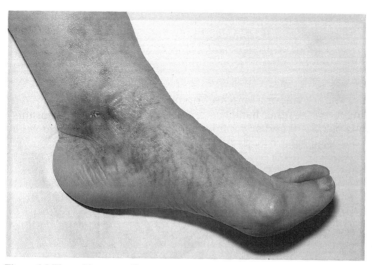

Figure 6.3 The ankle venous flare

phlebectatica[2], is the single most constant indication of calf perforating vein incompetence. Perforating vein incompetence is often described as the post-thrombotic syndrome and said to be characterised by secondary varices. While small local varicose veins are not infrequently found in the lower leg of patients with perforating vein incompetence, they are not by any means so common as the ankle venous flare. An ankle flare is a far more reliable indicator of perforating vein incompetence than 'fascial defects' palpated on the medial surface of the calf. Indentations in the subcutaneous superficial fat can often be felt, but these are more likely to represent superficial varices than defects in the deep fascia, and this is a most unreliable method of examination.

The next step in examining the veins of the lower limb is directed to the saphenous systems, long and short. In patients with varicose veins related to gross venous incompetence, the saphenous veins may be so dilated as to be obvious and no further examination or investigation is then necessary. In cases of doubt, and particularly in the obese patient, a number of simple tests and non-invasive investigations will determine whether these veins are normal or incompetent.

The groin cough impulse
This clinical test is mentioned first as it is the most commonly quoted in textbook accounts and is taught to all medical students. Unfortunately, it is no more reliable than attempting to detect perforating vein incompetence by palpating the skin of the lower leg. The cough impulse is certainly present in patients with a 'saphena varix', a large varix at the saphenofemoral junction. Unfortunately, this is by no means common. In the author's varicose vein clinic, a true saphena varix is present in no more than one in fifty of all patients with long saphenous incompetence. In the vast majority, the long saphenous vein, though dilated, is not grossly varicose, except perhaps in the lower thigh and upper calf; it is the tributaries of the saphenous veins which form most varicosities. For this reason, the cough impulse is not to be recommended as a test for saphenous incompetence, though when present it is an interesting physical sign.

The percussion test
This useful test was first described by Chevriér in 1908[3]. It is carried out in two steps.

1. The watching fingers are placed over the foramen ovale or the popliteal fossa, and the dilated saphenous vein, or a varicose tributary, in the lower leg is tapped briskly with the fingers of the other hand (Figure 6.4). The dilated vein transmits the pulse wave thus produced and an impulse can easily be felt by the watching fingers. Strictly speaking, the 'distal tapping, proximal watching' test only indicates a dilated vein and incompetence must be assessed by the second part of the test.
2. The reflux tapping test. The watching fingers and tapping fingers are now reversed. Tapping in the groin or popliteal fossa will produce a detectable impulse under the distal watching fingers if the vein is incompetent. It is arguable whether this part of the test is really necessary. While the first test strictly indicates dilatation rather than reflux, it is extremely rare for a competent saphenous vein (e.g. without reflux) to be sufficiently dilated for a tapping impulse to be detected proximally.

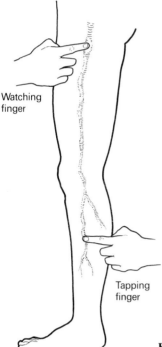

Watching finger

Tapping finger

Figure 6.4 The tapping test for saphenous incompetence

The percussion test can more easily be performed in obese patients by the addition of Doppler ultrasound. Instead of the pulse wave being detected by the watching fingers, the Doppler ultrasound probe is placed in the same position and the noise of the pulse wave can easily be heard in an incompetent and dilated vein.

The tourniquet test
This test was described by Trendelenburg in 1891[4]. The patient lies flat and elevates the leg. A tourniquet is applied at upper thigh or below knee level, depending on which saphenous vein is to be examined. Finger occlusion is often quicker and more accurate. The patient then stands and the leg is inspected to see whether the varices have been controlled. The tourniquet or finger is then suddenly released and the varices rapidly refill (Figure 6.5).

Like the previous test, this can be enhanced by the use of Doppler ultrasound[5]. With the patient standing, an obvious lower leg varix is marked with a felt-tip pen. The patient then lies, elevates the leg and the tourniquet is applied as before. The patient stands again and a Doppler ultrasound probe is placed over the marked point on the lower leg. When the tourniquet is suddenly removed, the rush of blood is detected by Doppler ultrasound and can be heard through its loudspeaker as a dramatic roaring noise, like a cascade of water. This modification is very useful in the excessively obese, where distal varices may be difficult to see and feel, and is also a most dramatic demonstration for students.

The author finds the groin cough impulse test of little value and the tourniquet test unnecessary except in the obese or in cases of doubt. The tapping test, with or

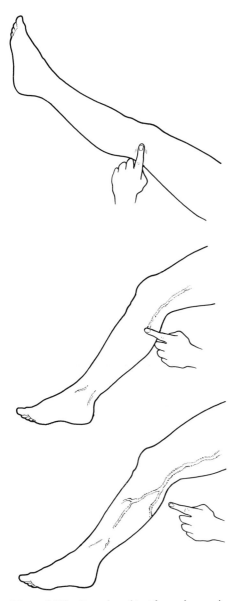

Figure 6.5 The 'tourniquet' test for saphenous incompetence. Either a tourniquet can be used or finger pressure as illustrated

without help from Doppler ultrasound, remains the mainstay of examination for saphenous incompetence. Like all tests performed in clinical examination, it requires practice, but this is easily attained in a busy varicose vein or ulcer clinic and an experienced examiner can usually detect the termination of the long or short saphenous vein with sufficient accuracy to enable the incision for its ligation to be performed precisely.

References

1. Negus, D. Calf pain in the post thrombotic syndrome. *Br. Med. J.* **2**: 156–158, 1968
2. Arnoldi, I. C., Haeger, K. Ulcus cruris venosum – crux medicorum? *Lakärtidningen* **64**: 2149–2157, 1967
3. Chevriér, L. De l'examin aux reflux veniaux dans les varices superficielles. *Arch. Gen. Chir.* **2**: 44–54, 1908
4. Trendelenburg, F. Über die Unterbildung der Vena saphena magna bi unterschenkel Variscen. *Beitr. Klin. Chir.* **7**: 195–210, 1891
5. Corbett, C. R. R., Parkhouse, N. How do you examine varicose veins? In *Phlebology '85* (eds Negus, D., Jantet, G.), London, Libbey, p. 113, 1986

Chapter 7

Diagnosis: methods of investigation

Recent developments in the non-invasive investigation of peripheral vascular disorders have provided the vascular surgeon with a profusion of new and useful techniques. These innovations may seem more confusing than helpful to those without previous experience of vascular laboratories. In this account therefore all the currently available methods will be described, with an indication of those the author personally finds most useful in the investigation of patients with leg ulcers and an indication of those instruments which should be obtained by those entering the field for the first time.

Investigation of the peripheral arteries and veins can be performed by both invasive and non-invasive methods. Invasive investigations include angiography and arterial and venous pressure measurements. Non-invasive methods include photoplethysmography, Doppler ultrasound, plethysmography (impedance, air or strain gauge), and ultrasound scanning, which may be combined with Doppler ultrasound flow detection in the Duplex scanner. The instruments can be used in a vascular laboratory, or most of them (photoplethysmography, Doppler ultrasound and strain gauge plethysmography) can be mounted on a mobile trolley (Figure 7.1), connected to a chart recorder or oscilloscope and used in the clinic. Non-invasive methods are most useful for initial rapid assessment and will therefore be described first.

Non-invasive investigations

Photoplethysmography

Photoplethysmography (PPG) depends on the emission and reflection of infra-red light (wavelength 805 nm). The instrument consists of a light-weight probe which contains both the light source and detecting crystal and this is attached to the skin by double-backed transparent adhesive tape. Light from the emitter is directed into the skin and the detector records changes in the intensity of the emergent light. In the AC mode, changes of blood flow enable the instrument to be used as a pulse recorder. For venous assessment a slow changing DC signal is used and this reflects changes in the volume of the subcutaneous venous plexus rather than pulsation.

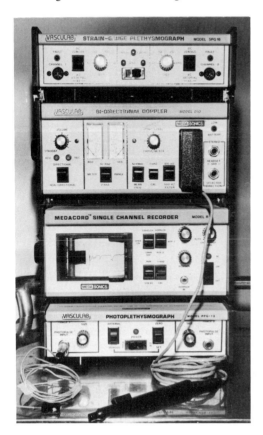

Figure 7.1 Photoplethysmograph, bidirectional Doppler ultrasound, single channel chart recorder and strain gauge plethysmograph. The diagnostic instruments can be connected to an oscilloscope and printer through a microcomputer, as an alternative to a chart recorder (Medasonics, California)

Arterial assessment

PPG in arterial mode is useful in assessing patients with suspected small vessel disease. In diabetes, or in patients with vasculitis, impaired perfusion of the toes and foot may be associated with normal pedal pulses and ankle pulse pressures (measured by Doppler ultrasound). The PPG probe is fixed to the pulp of the big toe by double-backed adhesive tape and the gain of the instrument is increased to provide maximum output. Pulse waves can be seen on a chart recorder or an oscilloscope similar to those produced by Doppler ultrasound (see Figure 7.4)' and, with a little experience, it is not difficult to distinguish between the sharply-peaked wave form of the adequately perfused toe from the damped and flattened wave form indicative of small vessel insufficiency. Quantitative assessment can be obtained by using small toe sphygmomanometer cuffs; the normal gradient between ankle pulse pressure and big toe pulse pressure is less than 30 mmHg.

Venous assessment

For venous assessment, PPG is used as follows.

With the patient sitting on a high stool, or on the edge of the examination couch (Figure 7.2), the probe is attached to the medial surface of the ankle above the

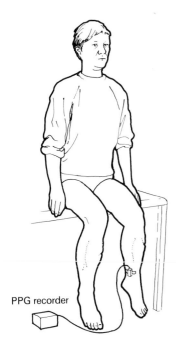

PPG recorder

Figure 7.2 Photoplethysmograph: venous assessment. Insert:
the probe is attached to the skin of the lower leg by
double-backed transparent adhesive tape

medial malleolus, care being taken to avoid placing it directly over the saphenous
vein, which will give a false reading. The trace on the chart recorder or oscilloscope
is adjusted to produce a baseline near the top of the chart paper or screen and, with
the recorder running, the patient is asked to move the ankle briskly up and down,
activating the calf muscle pump. The trace falls with each ankle movement as blood
is pumped out of the veins of the lower leg and the subcutaneous venular volume is
reduced, and the trace usually stabilises after five or six pumps of the calf muscle.

When the PPG trace is stabilised at its lower level, the patient is asked to stop
moving and relax and the time for the trace to return to baseline is noted. Venous
refilling time should normally be greater than 20 seconds, a more rapid recovery
time indicating some degree of venous incompetence (Figure 7.3). More rapid

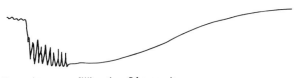

Normal trace: refilling time 34 seconds

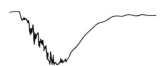

Venous reflux: refilling time 9 seconds

Figure 7.3 Photoplethysmograph. Top trace shows normal calf muscle pump, refilling time >20 seconds.
Lower trace shows venous reflux, refilling time <10 seconds

venous refilling will also sometimes occur in the normal leg if the investigation is performed in the late afternoon or in very hot weather. This should be remembered and PPG examination performed in the morning in cool conditions as far as possible. Comparison with foot venous pressure measurement has shown good correlation[1] but indeterminate results, with refilling times between 12 and 18 seconds, sometimes occur. These patients should be further investigated by foot venous pressure measurements and phlebography.

PPG can be used for more precise evaluation of the cause of venous incompetence by placing venous occlusion cuffs in various positions to occlude either the saphenous or perforating veins or both. Although this is sometimes useful, the results can be more difficult to interpret than those obtained by Doppler ultrasound, and the latter is preferable for detailed location of points of venous incompetence.

The most important feature of PPG is its ability to give a rapid assessment of venous calf muscle pump function. It is therefore most useful in patients presenting with oedema and in distinguishing oedema of venous origin from lymphoedema or cardiac or renal oedema. In fact ulceration is extremely uncommon in lymphoedema, and the presence of dorsal foot oedema in these patients usually makes the diagnosis obvious.

There are many surgeons who consider that the presence of deep venous incompetence contraindicates surgery for venous ulceration. PPG can be used to distinguish superficial from deep venous incompetence. If rapid refilling time persists in spite of control of the superficial veins by appropriate cuffs, deep venous incompetence can confidently be diagnosed and no operation is recommended. The author does not subscribe to this hypothesis and it is one of the purposes of this book to show that the presence of deep venous incompetence need not deter the surgeon from operating and that many ulcers in such patients can be healed by a combination of surgery and compression stockings. PPG is consequently less useful in the author's clinic than in the clinics of those who consider surgery contraindicated in the presence of deep venous incompetence.

Doppler ultrasound examination

Unlike PPG, whose chief value is in distinguishing the oedema of calf muscle pump failure from that of non-venous causes, Doppler ultrasound is the single most important instrument in the non-invasive evaluation of the ulcerated limb. A simple hand-held instrument is quite adequate, but the more complex instruments with zero crossing detection circuitry and output to a chart recorder or oscilloscope have a number of advantages, particularly in teaching. We use the Medasonics D10 instrument with two bidirectional pencil probes which have operating frequencies of 5 and 10 MHz. The former is suitable for venous investigations, the latter for arterial. These probes are bidirectional, a button on the probe allowing either forward or reverse flow to become dominant on the amplifier and thus enabling arterial pulsation to be damped out when examining veins. This is of considerable advantage, particularly in examination of the veins of the popliteal fossa.

Arterial assessment

Doppler ultrasound is invaluable in detecting pedal pulses, particularly in patients with venous oedema. Ankle pulses can easily be heard even when they cannot be

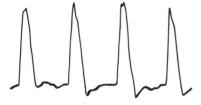

Figure 7.4 Doppler ultrasound: normal arterial pulsation

felt and wave forms can be visualised on the oscilloscope (Figure 7.4). Ankle pulse pressures can be measured by means of a sphygmomanometer cuff applied just above the probe. With the patient horizontal and the sphygmomanometer cuff in position, the flow probe is placed over the posterior tibial or dorsalis pedis artery and the cuff is inflated until the outflow signal ceases. During deflation of the cuff, a return of flow signal indicates the level of the systolic pressure at the ankle. Ankle pressures are compared to brachial systolic pressure measured at the same time and the ankle brachial pressure index should normally be greater than 1. An ankle systolic pressure of about 80–100 mmHg does not indicate severe reduction in skin blood flow, although such patients usually suffer from intermittent claudication. An ankle pressure of 70 mmHg or less is more usually found in patients whose ulcers are of ischaemic origin. A systolic pressure of less than 30 mmHg indicates very severe ischaemia which is unlikely to respond to sympathectomy.

A large or tender ulcer may make ankle pulse pressure measurement very difficult but this problem can be overcome in various ways. The cuff can be placed on the leg above the ulcer, though this is likely to result in an abnormally high pressure being recorded. Alternatively the ulcer can be covered with a dry dressing held in place with a light cotton bandage and the cuff placed over this. If both these manoeuvres are considered impossible, reliance must be placed on the Doppler signal. An experienced operator can get a good idea of pulse pressure simply by listening to the signal and distinguishing the sharp sound of a good systolic pulse wave from the slurred note of a damped wave. With the instrument connected to an oscilloscope or chart recorder on which the pulse wave can be observed, it is quite easy to tell whether this is suggestive of arterial insufficiency or not by the sharpness of the systolic peaks and the presence or absence of reversed flow. Doppler ultrasound can also be used for evaluating the popliteal pulse; the pulse pressure is measured by inflating a broad thigh cuff.

Evaluation of femoral artery blood flow is more difficult as no cuff can be applied above this point. An audible bruit over the femoral artery indicates stenosis, even if the arteriogram appears normal. As most atherosclerotic plaques in the iliac arteries lie on the posterior wall, an arteriogram film in the antero-posterior plane may well appear normal even in the presence of significant narrowing of the lumen. A crudely quantitative method of evaluating femoral artery blood flow has been described by Gosling et al.[2]. This method requires the use of a Doppler ultrasound apparatus which includes the measurement of mean velocity (this can be obtained electronically using the 0.1 Hz upper-frequency cut-off filter of the Hewlett-Packard Biolectric Amplifier, and is included in the Medasonics D10 instrument). Gosling has described a parameter called pulsatility index (PI), which is obtained by measuring the peak velocity of forward flow and that of reverse flow and dividing the difference in peak frequencies by the mean frequency. The same measurement is made on the aorta (or, in fat patients, on the brachial artery, on the assumption that there is no stenosis between the suprarenal aorta and the brachial artery), and the ratio of the proximal (brachial) PI to the distal (common femoral) PI is calculated. This is the damping factor (DF). A figure less than 1 indicates some degree of aortic or iliac stenosis. This is a relatively crude investigation, particularly as Skidmore et al.[3] have shown that an abnormal value does not distinguish between inflow stenosis and stenosis of the superficial femoral artery. A more accurate method of evaluating aortoiliac disease is by direct measurement of common femoral pressure combined with the use of papaverine and this is described under Invasive Methods.

Venous assessment

Venous occlusion

Doppler ultrasound can be used to detect venous occlusion by positioning the probe over the common femoral vein in the groin and squeezing the calf to produce a pulse wave. The patient should be positioned propped up at an angle of 45° with the ankle resting on a pillow so that the calf hangs free (Figure 7.5). This ensures

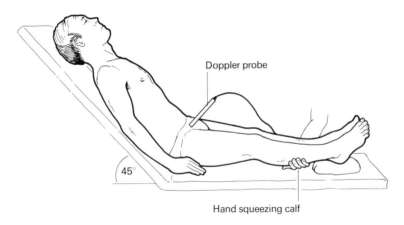

Figure 7.5 Doppler ultrasound examination for deep venous obstruction; note that patient's trunk should be elevated to ensure good filling of the calf sinusoids

maximal filling of the capacitance vessels in the calf and therefore a good pulse wave on compression (Figure 7.6). Patency of the iliac veins is assessed by asking the patient to take deep breaths or to perform a Valsalva manoeuvre; patent veins will transmit the respiratory swings to the common femoral vein where they are detected by the Doppler ultrasound probe. Venous occlusion is not common in the post-thrombotic ulcerated leg and this use of Doppler ultrasound is mainly of value in the early detection of acute deep vein thrombosis.

Venous incompetence

With the patient erect, the Doppler probe can be used to assess competence of each of the important systems: saphenous veins, the direct calf and ankle perforating veins and the popliteal and femoral veins.

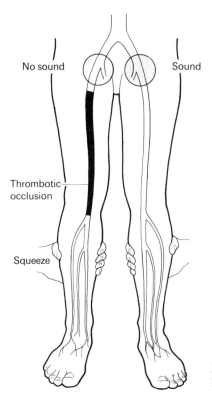

No sound

Sound

Thrombotic
occlusion

Squeeze

Figure 7.6 Doppler ultrasound assessment of deep vein patency

Saphenous veins   Examination for long saphenous incompetence by the modified Trendelenburg test using Doppler ultrasound has already been described. Long saphenous incompetence can also be detected by placing the Doppler ultrasound probe over the saphenous vein just below the saphenofemoral junction and listening for reflux after thigh squeezing. Examination for short saphenous reflux is carried out at the same time as examination for popliteal reflux and will be described under that heading.

Direct calf and ankle perforating veins   The fascial defects where these veins penetrate the deep fascia may be palpable in a thin leg and sometimes a small varix is visible at this point. Often there is no local varicosity and it is then that Doppler ultrasound is most useful. It is important that the patient is examined in the erect position to ensure maximal filling of the calf venous reservoir. A rough approximation of the site of an incompetent perforating vein can be obtained by observing the anterior and posterior borders of the ankle venous flare and extending these proximally to the point where the lines cross ('the coastal navigation sign') (Figure 7.7). The Doppler probe is then placed over this point and the observer's other hand repeatedly squeezes and releases the calf muscles at probe level (or the ankle or foot, distal to the probe) while the probe is moved slowly over the skin surface (Figure 7.8). A tourniquet is applied above the probe to exclude the effect of saphenous incompetence. Perforating vein incompetence is detected by a characteristic 'in and out' signal which is both audible and can be

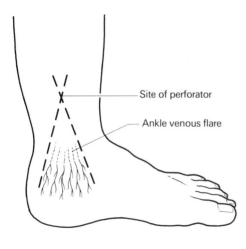

Figure 7.7 The 'coastal navigation' test for locating incompetent perforating vein. Extend the anterior and posterior borders of the ankle flare proximally and the perforating vein will be found close to where they cross

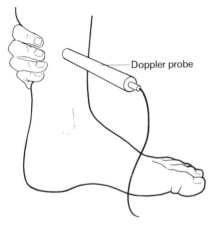

Figure 7.8 Doppler ultrasound detection of perforating vein incompetence

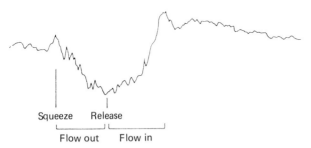

Figure 7.9 Doppler ultrasound trace showing inflow and outflow through an incompetent perforating vein

recorded (Figure 7.9). It should be emphasised that it is often impossible to carry out this examination satisfactorily in the presence of an infected or painful ulcer. Several weeks of ulcer cleaning and dressing may be necessary before examination is possible.

Femoral, popliteal and short saphenous veins Valvular competence of the superficial femoral, popliteal and short saphenous veins is assessed in similar manner by using the Doppler probe in the popliteal fossa. Maximal arterial pulsation is first found and the probe is then moved a little laterally. The calf is squeezed firmly (Figure 7.10) and proximal flow can be heard and observed on the oscilloscope or chart recorder. In the presence of normal valves in the popliteal and short saphenous veins, no retrograde flow is heard or observed on release of calf pressure (Figure 7.11). Valvular incompetence produces a distinct and prolonged

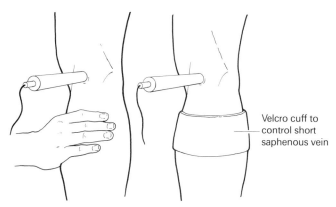

Figure 7.10 Doppler ultrasound investigation of popliteal and short saphenous incompetence; the cuff is used to occlude an incompetent short saphenous vein

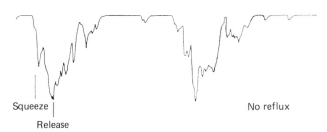

Figure 7.11 Doppler ultrasound trace demonstrating normal popliteal and short saphenous veins; forward flow only, no reflux

back flow signal (Figure 7.12a). Examination is much easier with the bidirectional probe, by means of which arterial pulsation can first be easily heard; by pressing the switch, flow along the femoral vein away from the probe is accentuated, and by pressing the switch again, reflux towards the probe can easily be heard. If reflux is present, it is important to distinguish short saphenous incompetence from popliteal incompetence. This is achieved by placing a narrow occlusion cuff around the upper calf, just below the popliteal fossa (Figures 7.10 and 7.12b). This will abolish reflux resulting from short saphenous incompetence but without popliteal incompetence. It is possible that reflux down incompetent gastrocnemial veins may mimic deep vein reflux but the condition is sufficiently rare for this potential error to be of little practical importance.

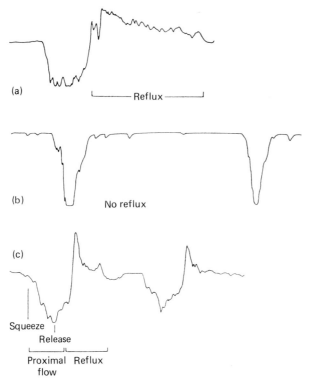

Figure 7.12 (a) Popliteal and/or short saphenous reflux. (b) Following compression cuff, no reflux, indicating short saphenous incompetence. (c) Reflux in spite of compression cuff indicates popliteal reflux

Other methods may be considered more useful in the evaluation of calf muscle pump function. While these are of interest to the physiologist or research surgeon, the clinician is more concerned with detecting signs of venous incompetence which may be amenable to surgical correction. Doppler ultrasound is outstandingly the most useful investigation for such detection and, in experienced hands, is similar to phlebography in accuracy[4].

Plethysmography

Limb volume changes can be used to evaluate limb blood flow, or, in the presence of constant arterial input, venous obstruction. Limb blood flow is very sensitive to changes in room temperature and a temperature-controlled room must be available. The technique is therefore usually limited to those with access to vascular laboratories in university hospital departments of physiology or surgery.

The original strain gauge plethysmographs consisted of mercury in rubber tubing, the resistance of which is directly proportional to the length. Nowadays indium–gallium alloy in Silastic tubing is more reliable and long-lasting (Figure 7.13). When placed around the calf, any change in the length of the gauge caused by a change in calf volume (and thus circumference) alters the resistance of the

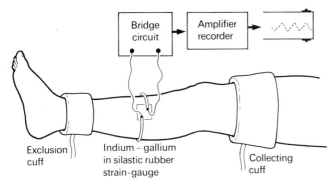

Figure 7.13 Strain gauge plethysmography

length of tubing and this in turn causes variations in the voltage drop across the gauge. The relative change in volume of the limb is equivalent to twice the relative change in its circumference (this is an approximation but sufficient for practical purposes)[5].

In the investigation of venous abnormalities, most usually of venous obstruction, there are now a number of plethysmographs available. These include phleborheography (PRG), strain gauge plethysmography (SPG), impedance plethysmography (IPG) and isotope plethysmography. For day to day clinical investigations, strain gauge plethysmography alone is sufficient and is useful in the non-invasive detection of pelvic venous obstruction. The rate at which blood flows out of the calf following venous congestion depends on the outflow resistance and also on the pressure gradient. The maximum venous otuflow, which is the rate of outflow in the first few seconds after venous congestion by a large pneumatic tourniquet round the thigh inflated to 50 mmHg for two minutes, can be used as a measure of proximal venous obstruction. An outflow less than 20 ml/100 ml/min is generally thought to indicate significant outflow obstruction. The method is insufficiently sensitive to detect minor obstruction caused by calf vein thrombosis but can be useful in the investigation of acute femoral vein thrombosis and chronic femoral or iliac venous stenosis or occlusion in cases of venous ulceration.

Strain gauge plethysmography can also be used in the investigation of venous reflux. Arterial inflow to the limb must first be occluded by a narrow cuff placed at the top of the thigh and inflated to 300 mmHg. A second, wide mid-thigh cuff is then rapidly inflated to 50 mmHg. In a normal limb, thigh cuff inflation expands the calf by 3%, whereas in a grossly incompetent venous system expansion may exceed 10%[6]. This is an uncomfortable test for the patient and is also of doubtful accuracy. The strain gauge plethysmograph can more simply be used to detect reflux by measuring venous refilling after erect exercise, but either photoplethysmography or foot volumetry are much more convenient methods and the strain gauge plethysmograph is best reserved for the detection of venous obstruction.

Individual sites of reflux (long or short saphenous vein, popliteal vein or perforating veins) can be detected by Doppler ultrasound. Doppler ultrasound, although probably less accurate than plethysmography, can also indicate the presence of venous obstruction, which can then be further investigated by ascending phlebography. In a fully equipped vascular laboratory, with experienced technical assistance, plethysmography is undoubtedly a useful investigation, but the beginner in this field, who is setting up a simple vascular assessment system in an ulcer clinic, should put plethysmography low on the list of purchases.

Foot volumetry

This modification of plethysmography was developed by Thulesius and his colleagues in 1973[7]. Whereas the conventional plethysmograph records changes in calf volume with the patient lying horizontally, foot volumetry consists of a temperature controlled water bath in which the patient stands. The water level changes with changes in foot volume and this can be measured electronically.

The foot is placed in the water bath and water at 32°C is added to a marked level on the bath wall. The volume of the foot is obtained by subtracting the volume of water added from the known volume of the bath. The patient holds on to a rail and performs twenty knee bends at one-second intervals. A normally-functioning calf muscle pump will pump blood from the foot and ankle, thereby reducing their volume, which results in a fall in the bath water level. The latter is precisely measured and recorded electronically. The patient then stands still and the rate of refilling or half-refilling is recorded.

This method enables measurement to be made of absolute expelled volume (EV), expelled volume relative to resting foot volume (EVr), refilling or half-refilling time, maximum rate of refilling and the ratio of maximum rate of refilling to relative expelled volume.

As with photoplethysmography, superficial and communicating veins can be controlled by tourniquets at various levels on the leg.

This is a valuable method in research, particularly in evaluating the effect of elastic compression stockings. It is less useful in clinical practice and the author does not use it in his vascular laboratory. The reasons for this are twofold. First, and most importantly, there must be some risk of cross-infection in patients with open ulcers. Secondly, like photoplethysmography, foot volumetry is not a good method of obtaining precise information about the points of reflux which are required to be controlled surgically in the treatment of venous ulceration. Doppler ultrasound examination and ascending venography are much more accurate in this respect.

Ultrasound imaging and Duplex scanning

B-mode ultrasound images are derived from the amplitude of the reflected ultrasound and the time it has taken to travel from the transmitting to the receiving crystals. Tissue density at known depths is reproduced as varying shades of grey, the so-called 'grey scale' image. The deep veins of the leg can be imaged using an 8 MHz probe above the knee and a 4 MHz probe below the knee. Obtaining a good image is more difficult than it might seem and, as in all other aspects of examination and investigation, experience is important. A skilled operator is able to detect floating or fixed thrombus and, in the post-thrombotic and ulcerated leg, the presence of reflux in the deep veins can be detected and incompetent perforating veins identified.

Duplex ultrasound is the combination of B-mode grey scale scanning with Doppler ultrasound flow detection and can be used to detect reduced blood flow in cases of thrombotic or post-thrombotic venous obstruction. The most recent development is the introduction of colour coding in which the computer identifies flow towards the probe and colours it red on the scan, flow away from the probe being coloured blue. This was initially used mainly in head and neck work to distinguish the carotid artery from the jugular vein, but is also useful in distinguishing arteries from veins in the lower limb, particularly in the popliteal fossa.

B-mode scanning should be available in the radiology department of all modern hospitals and the vascular surgeon setting up an ulcer clinic should discuss this with his radiologist and ensure that probes of the appropriate frequencies are available. Duplex and colour coded Duplex scanning are naturally more expensive but are likely to be available in teaching centres, particularly where much carotid artery surgery is carried out. If sophisticated apparatus is available, the vascular surgeon should make as much use of it as possible in the investigation of his ulcer patients. If Duplex scanning is not immediately available, it is probably not worth while going to a great deal of trouble and expense to obtain it, as a combination of other non-invasive investigations with modern venography should provide sufficient information about the underlying venous or arterial problem to enable effective treatment to be instituted.

This section has described currently available methods for the non-invasive investigation of patients with leg ulcers and has discussed their relative usefulness. In the next section, the invasive investigations of arteriography and venography are described. It is worth mentioning at this stage that, at the same time as these sophisticated non-invasive methods were being developed, there were parallel developments in radiological techniques and in improving contrast media. In arteriography, digital subtraction angiography has enabled the use of reduced volumes of contrast media and has also enabled visualisation of arteries through an intravenous injection. In venography, the conventional hyperosmolar contrast media, which were painful to the patient and whose use sometimes precipitated thrombosis, have now been replaced by low osmolar contrast media such as the non-ionic media iopamidol and iohexol. The clinician seeking to investigate the underlying cause of an ulcer need now be less concerned about the use of angiography, and a combined approach, using simple non-invasive methods, mainly photoplethysmography and Doppler ultrasound, with demonstration of the arterial or venous anatomy by angiography carried out by an expert, will provide sufficient information to enable effective treatment to be planned in nearly every case. At present, venography is usually necessary for accurate pre-operative assessment, *particularly in investigating disorders of the iliac veins*.

Invasive investigations

Invasive techniques for investigating the ulcer patient may be divided into two groups: (1) angiography, by which disordered anatomy may be displayed, and (2) pressure measurements to investigate disordered physiology.

Angiography
Huw Walters FRCR

Arteriography
Patients with leg ulcers accompanied by symptoms of arterial insufficiency, intermittent claudication or rest pain, or whose ankle pulse pressures are reduced,

may require investigation by arteriography. This is most commonly performed via the transfemoral route using local anaesthesia, a catheter being passed from the common femoral artery to the infra-renal abdominal aorta using the Seldinger technique. The arterial tree of both legs is then imaged by the injection of contrast medium and using a synchronised stepping table and cut-film changer. It must be remembered that haemodynamically significant iliac stenosis may not be seen in conventional arteriograms taken in the antero-posterior plane. Oblique films of the iliac arteries are sometimes helpful, as they are in detecting stenosis of the profunda origin, but aortoiliac pressure measurements are preferable in objectively evaluating the haemodynamic significance of an iliac stenosis (see below).

In investigating ulcerated legs it is particularly important to obtain arterial anatomy down to the ankle and foot, as occasionally ischaemic ulceration may occur as a result of quite localised arterial lesions.

Arterial flow in the lower limbs is unpredictable and often unequal in the presence of arterial disease. The timing of the radiographic exposure programme is important, and will often need to be tailored to the particular case to allow for this flow variation. To overcome this difficulty, a relatively large volume of contrast medium is injected at a slow rate (90 ml contrast medium at 10 ml/s) with an initial filming delay of 2.5 s from the commencement of the injection. Two radiographs are exposed at each of five consecutive and overlapping positions at a rate of one per second. This sequence is satisfactory in the majority of patients, and will demonstrate the full arterial tree from the aorta to the plantar arteries.

In occlusive vascular disease it is essential to visualise the full extent of the occluded segment(s) and to demonstrate the integrity of the vascular supply, both above and below the diseased vessel. Thus, with widely discrepant lower limb flow rates, delayed films are essential to demonstrate the more distal vessels after they have filled through collaterals. In this situation, having excluded aortoiliac 'inflow disease', as well as in those patients where problems are confined to one extremity, the injection of contrast is best made into the external iliac artery of the affected side, allowing a more controlled examination with a smaller volume of contrast medium. Where reconstructive surgery is planned below the knee, full arterial mapping to the plantar arch is required; in this situation lateral views of the calf may be useful in the evaluation of the tibial vessels. A close liaison with vascular surgical colleagues is ideal in planning the procedure to avoid arterial accessing in a groin where, in the short term, a possible vascular graft is planned on the basis of vascular laboratory studies. In this situation an approach from the contralateral femoral artery may be made, as also in the case of skin sepsis with infected groin lymph nodes.

Where both femoral arteries are impalpable, a translumbar aortogram (Figure 7.14) or a catheter study from a transaxillary approach may be undertaken if intravenous digital subtraction angiography is not available.

Venography

Patients presenting with venous ulceration confront the radiologist with an exacting challenge to display fully the vascular anatomy, thus allowing an accurate interpretation of the findings. In its basic form, venography involves the injection of contrast medium into one of the tributaries of the venous system, but requires a variety of special techniques to demonstrate veins in different regions, depending on the clinical presentation. The main variations of technique are in the method of

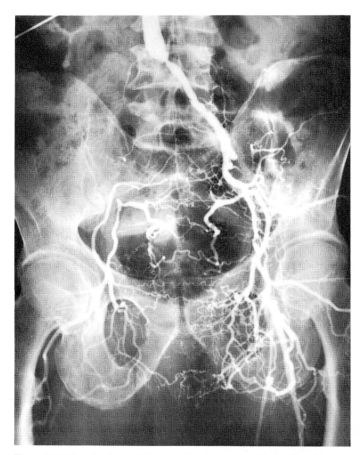

Figure 7.14 Translumbar arteriogram showing grossly atherosclerotic and occluded iliac arteries

introducing the contrast medium and in the postural and other manoeuvres designed to obtain uniform or selective venous filling.

A close clinical liaison with the vascular surgeon is essential so that the appropriate technique can be employed and the investigation tailored to answer the specific question arising from clinical examination, or queries arising from non-invasive vascular laboratory testing. Although there is a degree of overlap, non-invasive methods provide primarily functional information on the state of the veins whilst venography provides precise anatomical information. In many clinical situations, non-invasive methods and venography are complementary in providing specific information to enable effective surgical management.

Venographic techniques which may be employed in the investigation of patients presenting with leg ulceration include the basic ascending venogram, a modification of this basic study to demonstrate incompetent communicating veins, varicography, descending venography and iliocaval venography with pressure measurements. The basic equipment required is a radiographic tilting table equipped for fluoroscopy and with a spot-film capability. This system allows the direction of flow of contrast medium to be monitored and exposures made only when there is optimal venous filling. Iliocaval venography additionally requires an over-couch tube with a cut-film changer.

Basic ascending leg venogram

One of the most common indications for the basic ascending venogram in patients with venous ulceration is the demonstration of altered deep venous anatomy in those cases suspected, or shown, to have varying degrees of obstruction on non-invasive testing.

The patient is examined supine with a 20–40° foot-down table tilt. Table hand supports enable the patient to maintain position and avoid any weight-bearing on the leg under examination (Figure 7.15). The use of tourniquets, together with this semi-upright position, also promotes maximal and uniform filling of veins, thus avoiding flow artefacts.

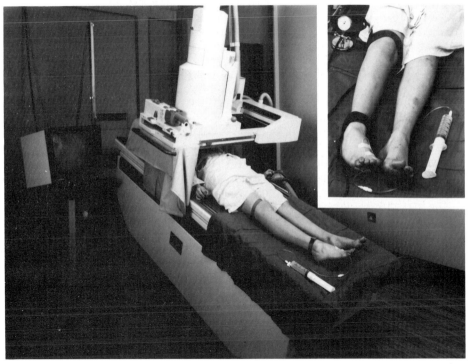

Figure 7.15 Fluoroscopy unit with the table in a 30° foot-down tilt. Hand grips provide support for this non weight-bearing position. The leg under examination (inset) is internally rotated to separate the images of the tibia and fibula

A self-fastening Velcro tourniquet is applied above the ankle to distend the foot veins. The skin on the dorsum of the foot is cleaned and a 21-gauge butterfly needle is inserted into a distal vein. Whilst any of these distal veins is acceptable, the medial digital vein of the great toe has the advantage of communicating directly, through the first interosseous space, with the plantar plexus. Injected contrast medium thus passes preferentially into the deep veins. The butterfly needle is secured and the venepuncture checked by injecting saline under direct vision.

A second tourniquet is applied above the knee to delay flow of contrast medium from the calf veins, serving also to promote more uniform filling of the deep distal veins.

The saline syringe is replaced with a syringe containing 60 ml of low osmolar contrast medium. The concentration routinely employed is 250 mg iodine/ml, and is obtained by diluting 50 ml iohexol 300 or iopamidol 300 with 10 ml saline. The volume of contrast medium required varies between patients, reflecting the differing venous capacity of legs. Optimal venous filling is determined by the appearances at fluoroscopy.

With the table in a 20–40° foot-down tilt and the leg under examination internally rotated to separate the images of the tibia and fibula, contrast medium is injected by hand under screen control. An injection rate of 0.5–1/ml is employed. The venepuncture site is checked to exclude extravasation, and the progress of the contrast medium is followed to ensure that it passes into the tibial veins. The ankle tourniquet pressure may require adjustment at this stage to ensure deep venous filling. The posterior tibial veins are normally the first to fill, followed by the fibular and anterior tibial veins. The muscular venous arcades of the soleus and gastrocnemius generally fill later than the main stem veins.

Films are exposed in the postero-anterior postion when there is uniform filling of the deep veins of the calf. Three exposures are made on a 35 cm × 35 cm radiograph, subdivided into three to include the veins from the ankle to the knee. Contrast filling of the popliteal venous segment is enhanced by gentle pressure of the deep calf veins just above the ankle. The leg is then externally rotated to obtain lateral views of the deep calf veins, three similar exposures being made to include the veins from the foot to the knee. These lateral views are important in demonstrating the posterior tibial veins and muscular venous arcades without superimposition of other veins.

The leg is now repositioned to the front and the above-knee tourniquet removed to allow contrast filling of the superficial and common femoral veins. Two exposures are made of the deep veins in the thigh. The explorator is finally positioned to include the area of the groin and pelvis. A third exposure is then made, following the release of the ankle tourniquet and the application of firm pressure to the calf to propel contrast medium as a bolus to demonstrate the iliac veins and lower inferior vena cava.

Following the procedure, and while the radiographs are being processed, the veins are cleared of contrast medium by leg elevation and injecting normal saline. Once the diagnostic adequacy of the examination is confirmed, early ambulation of the patient is encouraged. Possible thrombotic complications from stasis of the contrast medium are further reduced in this way.

The basic technique will demonstrate the extent of thrombotic occlusion, changes of recanalisation, collateral venous pathways and valvular damage or destruction. The resulting impaired function of the calf muscle pump results in the high pressure developed in the deep veins on exercise being transmitted through to the superficial veins via incompetent communicating veins (their localisation is described below).

During the procedure an indication of valvular incompetence secondary to post-thrombotic damage may be made by the performance of a Valsalva manoeuvre; venographically, however, descending venography provides a better test of valve function. Using a similar technique, short and long saphenous vein incompetence may be demonstrated when the popliteal and common femoral veins respectively are filled, the superficial veins then filling retrogradely. With short saphenous vein incompetence, a tourniquet applied above its termination will assist its demonstration when the vein fills in a retrograde direction. Radiographs in the lateral projection of the termination of the short saphenous vein are important because of the variation of anatomy in this region. Modification of the basic technique, with exclusion of the ankle tourniquet, may be required to demonstrate the variable termination of the short saphenous vein; alternatively, varicography may be of particular value, especially in recurrent cases. In some patients, this lateral projection will identify other venous tributaries, including incompetent gastrocnemius veins, which join the short saphenous or popliteal vein and may result in calf varices.

Modified basic technique to demonstrate incompetent communicating veins
Incompetent communicating veins play a major role in the aetiology of venous ulceration[4]. Precise information on their location is thus essential for effective surgical management.

Modification of the basic technique described above involves the selective delivery of contrast medium into the deep venous system, allowing identification of the site of these incompetent veins to be seen fluoroscopically as contrast passes retrogradely from the deep to the superficial veins. Pneumatic cuffs, as described by Craig[8], allow more efficient occlusion of the superficial veins at the ankle. The effectiveness of the ankle cuff can be checked on fluoroscopy. An above-knee cuff serves to delay the escape of contrast medium from the tibial veins, and assists in the demonstration of incompetent communicating veins.

The position of the ankle cuff may need to be modified and placed around the forefoot if ulceration is present at ankle level, or if an inframalleolar perforator is suspected. Further calf tourniquets may be required to occlude large incompetent communicating veins which allow excess filling of varicosities with contrast medium, since this degree of superficial venous filling may obscure more proximal incompetent veins.

The flow of the injected contrast medium is monitored and a radiograph exposed when retrograde flow through the incompetent vein is seen. These early films further aid identification of the precise level of the origin of the incompetent vein from the deep venous system, before excess superficial venous filling occurs. Localisation of the level of incompetent perforators can be measured by means of a ruler with 1 cm radio-opaque markers. This allows for magnification and the level is determined by reference to the malleoli (Figure 7.16).

Varicography
Varicography is the term applied to the technique of direct injection of contrast medium into varicose veins. Although described as a venographic technique nearly 40 years ago (Dow)[9], this method of investigation was not widely practised. This clinical lack of acceptance was almost certainly due to the high incidence of thrombotic complications which resulted from the injection of high osmolar contrast media into varicosities. The advent of the low osmolar contrast media, with a significantly reduced thrombotic potential[10], has resulted in a wider application of a valuable technique, particularly in the investigation of recurrent varicose veins.

The patient is first examined in the erect position to optimally display the varicose network of veins. A 21-gauge butterfly needle is introduced into a suitable

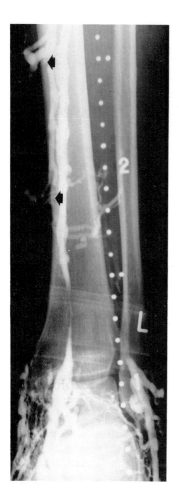

Figure 7.16 Ascending venogram with effective ankle tourniquet pressure allowing selective deep venous filling. An early exposure allows identification of incompetent veins (black arrows); their level is determined from the 1 cm radio-opaque markers

vein in this symptomatic varicose complex. With the needle secured, the patient lies on the fluoroscopy table in either the prone or supine position, depending on the position of the needle.

The fluoroscopy table is positioned to a 10–20° foot-down tilt, and the flow of contrast medium is monitored to determine the direction of drainage of the varicosities through the perforating veins to the deep venous system. With varicosities in the short saphenous territory, a lower thigh tourniquet, applied above the saphenopopliteal junction, will retard the flow of contrast away from the popliteal vein and enhance the filling of incompetent veins in relation to both the short saphenous and popliteal veins. Lateral projections are essential in this situation to display adequately the variable anatomy which may be found at the saphenopopliteal junction (Figure 7.17). The filling of hunterian and other thigh perforating veins is similarly enhanced with the placement of a tourniquet above the incompetent vein. Lateral views are also helpful with hunterian perforators to allow accurate localisation in two planes. A ruler with opaque distance markers allows for magnification, and the level is determined by reference to the femoral condyles.

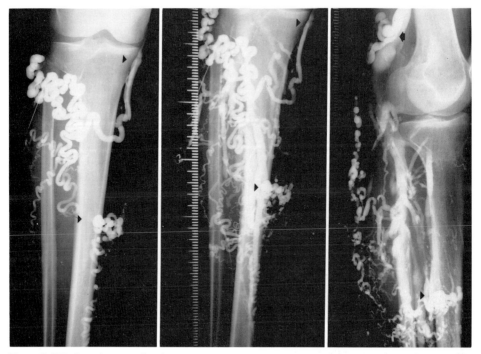

Figure 7.17 Left: varicogram showing complex recurrent varicose network communicating medially with long saphenous varicosities (arrowheads). Centre: deep venous filling is present, due to perforator (lower arrowhead) at this level. Right: lateral view showing communication with recurrent short saphenous varicosities (arrow)

In the long saphenous territory, varicose vein recurrences may arise from the groin, or more distally through incompetent communicating veins between the deep system and any part of the long saphenous vein not identified at surgery (Figure 7.18). It is therefore of considerable importance to determine the site of recurrence to avoid a possible abortive re-exploration in an area distorted by previous surgery. Varicography is initially undertaken with the fluoroscopy table tilted foot-down and, as the contrast injection is continued, the table is moved through into a 30–40° head-down position. Table hand supports provide a secure position for the patient. Spot films are made to record the central deep venous communications.

Varicography may however fail to demonstrate the full extent of recurrent groin varices, since contrast medium under gravity in the head-down table tilt position will tend to follow the path of least resistance. Descending venography with a Valsalva manoeuvre will however distend the varices and demonstrate their full extent[11]. This technique is described below.

Descending venography
Descending venography was originally applied in the evaluation of the competence or otherwise of the valves in the deep veins. The procedure involves the placement of a 19-gauge Potts Cournand needle (Becton Dickinson, Rutherford, NJ) into the common femoral vein under local anaesthesia. The examination is carried out with the patient in the erect or steep semi-erect position. Contrast medium is injected

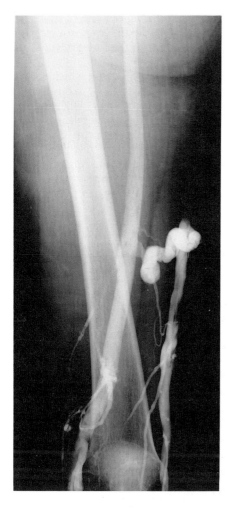

Figure 7.18 A large Hunterian incompetent communicating vein not identified at surgery. The long saphenous vein had been ligated just proximal to the incompetent vein

slowly by hand in 15–20 ml boluses. The progress of the contrast is monitored fluoroscopically and spot films made to record the extent of retrograde flow. A Valsalva manoeuvre may assist the retrograde flow of contrast as far as competent valves allow, but the erect position is usually adequate. Some reflux of contrast medium is normal due to gravity and the density of the medium. Reflux to the knee or below is however abnormal, and the damaged valves will be apparent.

Reference has already been made to the possible application of descending venography in some patients with recurrent groin varices.

Iliocaval venography
Iliac vein thrombosis frequently fails to recanalise with maturation, and a permanent occlusion may result. When recanalisation does occur, the vein is often narrowed with stenotic segments. Collateral venous pathways then develop and iliac venography will demonstrate these collateral pathways. The development of these venous collaterals may be sufficient to compensate for the iliac vein stenosis

or occlusion, so that no functional obstruction results to the venous return from the leg. Pressure measurements, as described below, are essential to evaluate the functional significance of these occlusions/stenoses, and are an integral part of iliocaval venography[12].

The patient is examined in the supine position on a fluoroscopy unit which is also equipped with an over-couch tube and cut-film changer. Two 19-gauge cannulas are introduced, one in each common femoral vein, under local anaesthesia. Venepuncture is facilitated by the patient performing a Valsalva manoeuvre to distend the femoral vein. Test injections of contrast medium confirm correct needle placement. Low osmolar contrast medium (40 ml) is then simultaneously injected into the common femoral veins by two operators. The injection rate must be such as to deliver the volume in 4–5 s. The filming sequence is commenced at the same time as the injection, eight exposures being made at the rate of one per second using a serial film changer.

A single spot film would serve to demonstrate any occlusion but serial exposures allow a better display of the altered anatomy, demonstrating the extent and direction of flow through venous collaterals (Figure 7.19).

Where the femoral vein is occluded, the proximal extent of the occlusion can be defined by one of three alternative approaches: retrograde iliac venography where the contralateral femoral vein is patent; descending retrograde iliocavography via a catheter introduced from a median antecubital vein; or by pertrochanteric intraosseous venography, which however requires a general anaesthetic.

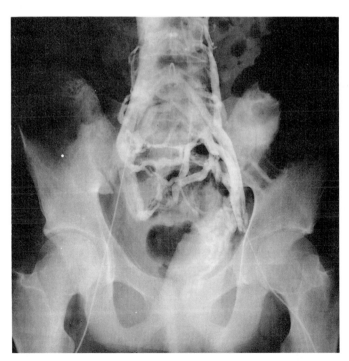
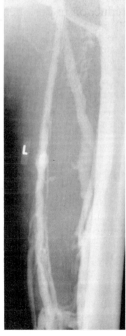

Figure 7.19 Left: post-thrombotic occlusion of the left common iliac vein with established collaterals through the pre-sacral plexus, ascending lumbar vein and developing pudendal collaterals. Right: ascending venogram also showed post-thrombotic changes in the superficial femoral vein and external iliac vein.

At completion of the procedure, the femoral vein pressures are taken at rest and following exercise, as described below.

Pressure measurements

Arterial pressure measurements

The difficulty of detecting and quantifying stenoses in the aorta or iliac vessels has been discussed in the section on non-invasive investigations. It is most important to exclude haemodynamically significant iliac or aortic stenosis when considering the suitability of a patient for femoropopliteal bypass grafting. A stenosis, which may not be visible on conventional arteriography, may still reduce blood flow to the graft to an extent sufficient to cause early graft thrombosis. Calculation of the pulsatility index and damping factors can provide a crude assessment but more accurate information can be obtained by direct cannulation of the femoral artery, either at the same time as angiography or at the start of a surgical exploration. Femoral artery pressure can be compared with the pressure in the distal aorta by passing the cannula through the stensosed iliac vessels to the infrarenal aorta. Alternatively, comparison can be made with the brachial systolic pressure measured simultaneously. Measurements should be performed at rest and also following hyperaemia. The latter can either be induced by applying a thigh cuff to occlude the blood supply of the limb for three minutes (release of this tourniquet results in reactive hyperaemia) or alternatively papaverine sulphate can be injected through the cannula in the common femoral artery[13]. Limb hyperaemia and reduction in peripheral resistance causes a drop in femoral arterial pressure if the iliac arteries are patent.

Venous pressure measurements

In the evaluation of peripheral venous incompetence, foot venous pressure measurements and their response to exercise are a long-established procedure. Femoral venous pressure measurement is indicated in the investigation of suspected iliac obstruction.

Foot venous pressure measurement
This method of evaluating venous function was first described by Beecher and his colleagues in 1936[14]. The introduction of the pressure transducer has improved the sensitivity of the investigation. It is generally considered a more accurate method of evaluating calf muscle pump function than either photoplethysmography, strain gauge plethysmography or foot volumetry. By cannulating the long saphenous vein on the dorsum of the foot, close to its communication with the plantar veins through the foot perforating veins, foot venous pressure measurement can be used as a test both of saphenous incompetence and of deep venous incompetence. Where the two co-exist, occlusion of the saphenous vein by a tight ankle cuff results in foot venous pressure changes being related to the state of the deep veins.

Foot venous pressure measurement is performed by cannulating a suitably large vein on the dorsum of the foot; the cannula is then connected to a strain gauge manometer sensitive enough to detect changes of 2–5 mmHg. The pressure transducer is placed at the level of the cannula and the patient stands perfectly still until the foot venous pressure rises to a height equivalent to the distance between the foot and the right atrium (see Figures 4.2 and 4.3). The patient then exercises by raising both heels off the ground and, with a normal calf muscle pump, the foot venous pressure progressively falls until it stabilises at about 25 mmHg after five or six calf muscle contractions. The patient then again stands still and the time taken for the trace to return to baseline is observed. This is normally between 25 and 30 seconds.

The exercising fall in pressure indicates the efficiency of calf muscle pump function, and a decrease in venous refilling time indicates reflux. Information about the site of reflux can be obtained by applying appropriate occlusion cuffs.

The criticism against dorsal foot venous pressure measurement is that venous ulceration is rarely if ever seen on this site (dorsal foot ulcers are usually ischaemic in origin), while venous ulcers do occur on the medial surface of the ankle, whose venous drainage is primarily through the perforating veins. It can be argued that the photoplethysmograph, being placed on the medial surface of the ankle in the region of the ankle flare veins, is more likely to reflect direct perforating vein incompetence, which is primarily responsible for venous ulceration.

Foot venous pressure measurement is still considered the most accurate method for use in experimental laboratories. In our ulcer clinic however we find that sufficient information about the state of the superficial, perforating and deep veins can nearly always be obtained by a combination of photoplethysmography, Doppler ultrasound examination and ascending venography, and foot venous pressure measurement is very rarely necessary.

Femoral venous pressure measurement
Femoral venous pressure studies must always be performed in the investigation of suspected iliac vein stenosis (Figure 7.20). Apparent stenosis shown on iliac venography may not in fact be sufficient to obstruct venous return. On the other hand, iliac vein occlusion, usually at the junction of the left common iliac vein and the inferior vena cava, may be sufficiently compensated by the development of adequate venous collaterals, so that there is no functional obstruction to venous return from the leg (see Figure 3.12, page 25).

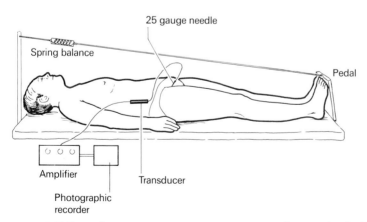

Figure 7.20 Femoral venous pressure measurement at rest and on exercise. In this sketch of our original studies, constant counter-pressure was applied to the foot by means of a spring balance. This is not necessary in practice but the foot should press against some form of resistance in order to ensure maximum muscle contraction

A saline manometer is perfectly adequate for this measurement, though a pressure transducer will enable a permanent record to be made. With the patient lying supine and horizontally, the common femoral vein is cannulated under local anaesthetic. There is normally no difference in resting pressure between right and left sides and this pressure is normally between 8 and 10 mmHg[9]. Resting pressures alone are inadequate to demonstrate obstruction to blood flow which must be increased by exercising the limb. The patient is asked to perform energetic foot movements of the affected leg against resistance. The exercising femoral venous pressure in a patient with patent iliac veins and a patent vena cava does not rise more than 2 mmHg. Resistance due to proximal stenosis results in a rise in pressure of up to 18 mmHg (Figure 7.21). Observing exercising as well as resting venous

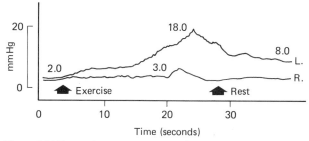

Figure 7.21 Femoral venous pressure measurement in a patient with post-thrombotic left iliac occlusion. When the pressure reached 18 mmHg, the patient complained of severe 'bursting' calf pain and was no longer able to continue exercising the leg

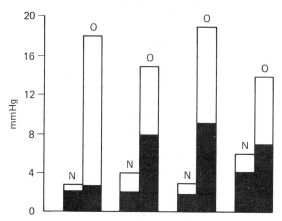

Figure 7.22 Histogram of resting (■) and exercising (□) femoral venous pressures (supine) in four patients with post-thrombotic obstruction of one iliac vein. N, normal; O, obstructed

pressures accentuates the effect of any stenosis and is also useful in the unusual situation of bilateral iliac or inferior vena cava occlusion. A positive diagnosis of significant proximal venous obstruction can be made if the exercising pressure rise is greater than 2 mmHg and there is no absolute need to compare the resting pressure in one leg with that in the other (Figure 7.22).

Priorities in the investigation of leg ulcers

In this chapter the methods of investigation which should be available in a fully equipped modern vascular laboratory have been described. The clinician who is only interested in obtaining essential information on which to diagnose the underlying cause of leg ulceration has no need of such complicated and expensive equipment. The most useful investigations have been indicated in this chapter and, for quick reference, a suggested list of priorities is given below.

Non-invasive investigations

1. *Doppler ultrasound* (inexpensive hand held instrument is adequate): essential for arterial pulse detection in oedema, arterial pulse pressures, saphenous and popliteal reflux, detection of incompetent perforating veins.
2. *Photoplethysmography*: very useful, particularly in distinguishing oedema of venous origin from non-venous causes.
3. *Strain gauge plethysmography*: not essential but very useful for diagnosing venous obstruction.
4. *Foot volumetry* (Thulesius water bath): useful in research (e.g. effectiveness of stockings) but more convenient for the non-ulcerated leg. The author does not personally use this investigation.
5. *Duplex scanning*: not essential for the ulcer clinic vascular laboratory but ideally patients should have access to Duplex scanning; can be most helpful in evaluating femorofemoral graft patency and also peripheral venous obstruction and reflux.

Invasive methods

1. *Angiology – arteriography and venography*: essential, most important to have access to a radiologist with experience in venography.
2. *Femoral artery pressure measurement*: important in excluding proximal stenosis in patients considered for femoropopliteal bypass grafting.
3. *Foot venous pressure measurement*: not essential; photoplethysmography may not be so precise but, combined with Doppler ultrasound and venography, provides sufficient information for clinical management.
4. *Femoral venous pressure measurement*: essential in the diagnosis of the iliac occlusion requiring surgical correction.

References

1. Flynn, W. R., Queral, L. A., Abramowitcz, H. B., *et al*. Photoplethysmography in the assessment of chronic venous insufficiency. In *Investigation of Vascular Disorders* (eds Nicolaides, A. N., Yao, J. S. T.), New York, Churchill Livingstone, 1981
2. Gosling, R. G., Dunbar, G., King, D. H., *et al*. The quantitative analysis of occlusive peripheral arterial disease by a non-obstructive ultrasonic technique. *Angiology* **22**: 52–55, 1971
3. Skidmore, R., Woodcock, J. P., Wells, P. N. T., Bird, D., Baird, R. N. Physiological interpretation of Doppler-shift waveforms. III. Clinical results. *Ultrasound Med. Biol.* **6**: 227–231, 1980
4. Negus, D., Friedgood, A. The effective management of venous ulceration. *Br. J. Surg.* **70**: 623–625, 1983
5. Whitney, R. J. Measurement of volume changes in human limbs. *J. Physiol. (Lond.)* **121**: 1–27, 1953

6. Barnes, R. W., Collicott, P. E., Mozersky, D. J., Sumner, D. S., Strandness, D. E. Jr. Non-invasive quantitation of venous reflux in the post-phlebitic syndrome. *Surg. Gynecol. Obstet.* **136**: 769–773, 1973

7. Thulesius, O., Norgren, L., Gjores, J. E. Foot volumetry, a new method for objective assessment of edema and venous function. *Vasa* **2**: 325–329, 1973

8. Craig, J. O. In *Practical Procedures in Diagnostic Radiology,* 2nd edn (eds Saxton, H. M., Strickland, B.), London, H. K. Lewis, p. 250, 1972

9. Dow, J. D. The venographic diagnosis of the method of recurrence of varicose veins. *Br. J. Radiol.* **25**: 382, 1952

10. Walters, H. L., Clemenson, J., Browse, N. L., Lea Thomas, M. ^{125}I-fibrinogen uptake following phlebography of the leg. *Radiology* **135**: 619–621, 1980

11. Lea Thomas, M., Phillips, G. W. Recurrent groin varices: an assessment by descending phlebography. *Br. J. Radiol.* **61**: 294–296, 1988

12. Negus, D., Cockett, F. B. Femoral vein pressures in post-phlebitic iliac vein obstruction. *Br. J. Surg.* **54**: 522–525, 1967

13. Udoff, E. J., Barth, K. H., Harrington, D. P., *et al.* Haemodynamic significance of iliac artery stenosis. Pressure measurements during angiography. *Radiology* **132**: 289–293, 1979

14. Beecher, H. K., Field, M. E., Krogh, L. The effect of walking on the venous pressure of the ankle. *Scand. Arch. Physiol.* **73**: 133, 1936

Chapter 8

The differential diagnosis of leg ulcers

The successful treatment of ulcers depends on accurate diagnosis, which itself depends on the examination and investigations described in Chapters 6 and 7. As in all branches of clinical medicine, experience is helpful, but a spot diagnosis can often be inaccurate and the sensible clinician will arrange confirmatory investigations, even when he is 90% sure of the underlying cause of the ulcer. Most leg ulcers seen in the UK are venous or ischaemic in origin. Infectious ulcers are more commonly seen in tropical countries; neoplastic ulcers are rare, but it is most important always to be aware of this possibility and there are a number of less common causes which are difficult to classify.

Venous ulcers

Ulceration related to local varicosity

The true varicose ulcer, that is an ulcer related entirely to superficial varicosity arising from saphenous incompetence and reflux, is rare. Careful examination of patients with varicose veins and ankle ulceration will usually demonstrate perforating vein incompetence.

Site and appearance
Varicose ulcers usually occur on the anterior or lateral surface of the lower leg or ankle rather than in the malleolar regions. They may occur anywhere on the lower leg or ankle; their one constant feature is that they are invariably related to a large dilated varicose vein (Figure 8.1). Varicose ulcers are usually small, shallow and painless, with a well-epithelialised edge and a base of healthy granulation tissue. They often arise in an area of varicose eczema.

History and examination
The patient will usually have a long history of primary varicose veins, often with a similarly affected parent. There is unlikely to be any history of deep vein thrombosis. The most common complaint is of aching legs on prolonged standing, sometimes with ankle oedema. Night cramps are common and a few patients complain of severe burning pain in the feet; it is important to exclude a peripheral neuropathy in such patients.

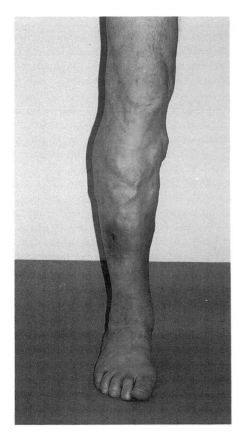

Figure 8.1 Varicose ulcer: small, anterior surface of leg, overlying varix

Examination will show large calf and ankle varices, most usually arising from a grossly distended long saphenous vein. This can be confirmed by the percussion and tourniquet tests. The latter is often helpful in fat patients. There may be patches of varicose eczema. Peripheral ischaemia must be excluded by careful palpation of the ankle pulses, augmented by Doppler ultrasound if this examination leaves any doubt. Examination of the ankle should not show a venous flare in a case of true varicose ulceration. Doppler ultrasound should be used to exclude calf perforating vein incompetence and also popliteal incompetence.

Venography is usually unnecessary, though varicography may be indicated if the varicose veins are recurrent, when it is important to demonstrate their site of communication with the deep system.

Ulceration related to perforating/deep venous incompetence

The original description of post-phlebitic ulceration has now been largely abandoned as many patients with chronic liposclerosis and ankle ulceration have no history of deep vein thrombosis. The term 'venous ulcer' is less specific and allows a variety of causes.

Site and appearance

Venous ulcers are most commonly found over the medial malleolus (see Figure 5.3), less commonly over the lateral malleolus, and occasionally these ulcers may meet posteriorly or even become completely circumferential. They vary in depth from 1 or 2 mm to extending down to the deep fascia. They are almost always much deeper than varicose or vasculitic ulcers.

Venous ulcers are almost invariably accompanied by an ankle venous flare of fine superficial venules and usually by pigmentation and lipodermatosclerosis. These physical signs are likely to be seen accompanying smaller ulcers; very large ulcers may include all the skin normally occupied by the venous flare or liposclerosis (Figure 8.2).

Most venous ulcers are infected when the patient first presents to the clinic and the ulcer base may be obscured by purulent debris and slough. Once this has been removed the base is seen to consist of healthy pink granulation tissue. If this is not obviously pink, suspect ischaemia. The ulcer edge is also pink and slopes gently to the ulcer base. The edge may be punched out in an infected ulcer but this appearance should rapidly change following appropriate treatment. Undermined edges suggest tuberculosis or other chronic infection.

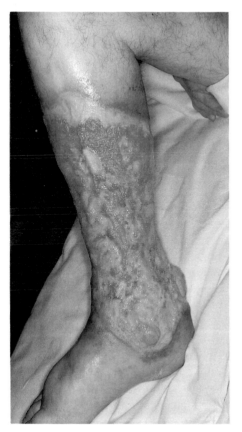

Figure 8.2 Gross venous ulceration; this patient eventually required amputation

History
A history of local trauma is common. In the days of bus conductors, elderly ladies often fell on the bus step when it moved off unexpectedly. Now that buses are mostly single-manned, the supermarket trolley is mainly responsible for similar trauma. A past history of deep vein thrombosis is common but not universal. In the Lewisham Hospital series, only 45 of 77 patients with 109 ulcerated legs (58%) gave a history of previous deep vein thrombosis.

If the patient gives a history of previous iliofemoral thrombosis, particularly in the left leg, there may be chronic iliac vein occlusion with obstruction to venous outflow from the limb. The patient should be asked whether he or she has experienced any calf swelling (as opposed to ankle oedema, which is common in varicose veins and perforating vein incompetence) and, most importantly, whether there are any symptoms suggestive of venous claudication. This is severe calf pain (sometimes described as 'bursting' in nature), which occurs on walking 100 or 200 metres[1]. This is much more severe than the dull ache on prolonged standing experienced by many patients with venous incompetence.

Examination
Examination of the limb with venous ulceration has two main purposes: firstly to identify all points of venous reflux and possible venous obstruction, and secondly to exclude arterial insufficiency as a contributory factor.

The patient is first examined lying flat and the site and appearance of the ulcer is noted. Particular note is taken of the presence or absence of surrounding lipodermatosclerosis and also whether an ankle venous flare is visible. The latter is usually present and indicates direct calf perforating vein incompetence, but may be completely obscured by a very large ulcer. Signs of iliac vein obstruction are looked for, small dilated groin collateral veins, and an increase in calf circumference on the affected side (see Figure 6.1). Abdominal and rectal examination must be performed in all patients with a swollen limb.

With the patient standing on an 18 cm (7 in) mounting block, the leg is re-examined after a delay of about 30 seconds to allow for venous filling. The presence of varicose veins is noted and their communication with long or short saphenous systems identified by examination and the percussion and tourniquet tests, as necessary. An ankle venous flare may become more obvious in the erect position.

The patient's toes and forefoot must be examined for evidence of ischaemia, e.g. cyanosis and slow capillary refilling time. Ankle and foot pulses must be palpated. Doppler ultrasound examination may be necessary if these are obscured by oedema.

Investigations
Doppler ultrasound examination may be helpful in identifying long saphenous incompetence, as indicated in Chapter 6, but its chief value is in identifying sites of perforating vein incompetence and also popliteal and short saphenous incompetence. It has been taught that incompetent perforating veins can be identified by 'feeling the defect in the deep fascia'. This is an extremely unreliable method of examination; most of these supposed fascial defects are in fact indentations in the superficial fat related to dilated varices. Doppler ultrasound is a far more reliable method of identifying perforating vein incompetence and its use has been described in Chapter 7, page 64. Its use in identifying popliteal or short saphenous incompetence has also been described in that chapter.

If deep venous obstruction is identified, this can also be quickly evaluated by Doppler ultrasound, as has been described. Doppler ultrasound is also useful in detecting pulses which may be difficult to palpate due to ankle oedema.

Strain gauge plethysmography is useful in investigating possible proximal venous obstruction, and this is described on page 71.

Duplex scanning, if available, can be used to investigate popliteal and saphenous reflux, perforating vein incompetence and proximal venous obstruction.

Venography   Ascending venograms (Figure 8.3) are usually necessary in order to provide more precise information about the site of incompetent perforating veins than is possible with non-invasive methods, and venography is also useful in demonstrating deep venous recanalisation, stenosis or occlusion. Venographic evidence of iliac vein occlusion must be further investigated by femoral venous pressure measurements at rest and on exercise (see page 84), as venography alone cannot evaluate the effectiveness of the collateral venous circulation in bypassing the obstructed iliac vein.

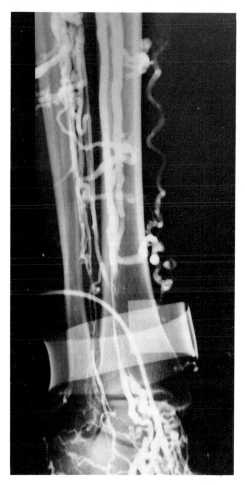

Figure 8.3 Ascending venogram: incompetent direct perforating vein communicating with superficial veins

Ischaemic ulceration

Site and appearance

Ischaemic ulcers may be situated on the toes or forefoot in an area of cyanosed and obviously pregrangrenous skin. Another common site is the heel, particularly in bed-ridden patients. These ulcers are usually accompanied by severe rest pain and there is no difficulty in making a diagnosis.

Ischaemic ulcers may also present on the dorsum of the foot or on the anterior surface of the leg or may mimic venous ulcers by being situated over the medial or lateral malleolus. The latter are often no more painful than venous ulcers and the diagnosis is then by no means easy.

The base of a typical ischaemic ulcer is usually obscured by pale yellow purulent exudate and necrotic debris, often with islands of gangrenous skin. Removal of the necrotic debris is likely to reveal deep fascia or tendon, with little or no granulation tissue. The edges are very poorly epithelialised and may be punched out (Figure 8.4).

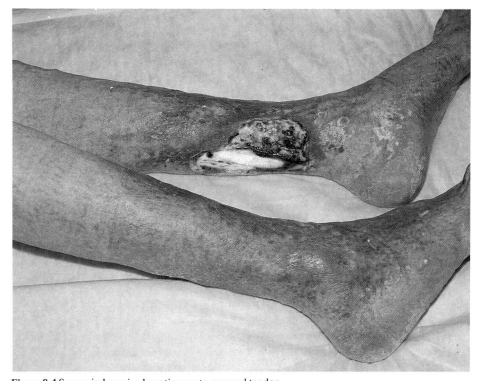

Figure 8.4 Severe ischaemic ulceration; note exposed tendon

History

A history of ischaemic rest pain is common in the more severe cases and lesser degrees of ischaemia are usually associated with intermittent claudication. The patient is often a heavy cigarette smoker. Many patients are very old and bed-ridden. This is particularly true of heel ulcers, which are usually described as pressure sores. Conscientious ward sisters often become upset when these occur as they are considered an indication of inadequate nursing. While this may sometimes be true, the blood supply of the heels of these old people is often so severely reduced that the skin will break down in spite of efforts to prevent pressure.

Examination and investigations
Ischaemic ulceration usually occurs in an area of obviously ischaemic skin, which may be cyanosed or pale and shiny. All pulses must be palpated: femoral, popliteal and ankle pulses. Oedema may make the last difficult to feel, in which case Doppler ultrasound should be used. It is not sufficient simply to palpate one ankle pulse, for instance the dorsalis pedis, and then assume that there must be adequate arterial perfusion of the lower leg and foot. The author has seen three patients with ankle ulceration in whom only one ankle pulse could be palpated. In each case, the ulcers healed satisfactorily following chemical lumbar sympathectomy. The ankle pulse pressures of diabetic patients with ischaemic ulceration may appear normal or abnormally high. This is due to increased stiffness of the walls of small arteries in diabetes, which makes pulse pressure measurement unreliable. Ischaemic ulcers can also result from small vessel insufficiency, particularly in diabetes, thromboangiitis obliterans (Buerger's disease) and the vasculitides. Ankle pulse pressures may then be normal and diagnosis depends on examination of the toe capillary refilling time and on the measurement of toe pulse pressures using PPG and a miniature sphygmomanometer cuff. The pressure gradient between ankle and toes should not normally exceed 30 mmHg.

Arteriography is mandatory, except in the elderly who are unfit for direct arterial surgery and whose ulcers respond to lumbar sympathectomy or prostacyclin infusion.

Case report
A 56-year-old man was referred to the Lewisham Hospital vascular clinic with a letter asking for treatment of the 'venous ulcer' over his left medial malleolus. This had been treated by tight medicated compression bandaging for two years and his doctor felt that failure to heal required a second opinion. Examination showed a shallow ulcer over the medial malleolus. There was no obvious evidence of venous abnormality but further examination also showed that his second and third toes had been amputated and the amputation site was ulcerated and obviously ischaemic.

Further questioning revealed that this patient had been involved in an accident some five or six years previously and this had been followed by the amputation of two toes. He said that the amputation site had failed to heal and he was subsequently referred to a vascular clinic elsewhere for lumbar sympathectomy. Temporary healing was followed by further breakdown and then development of the ankle ulcer.

Neither femoral pulse could be palpated and arteriography demonstrated atherosclerotic occlusion of both iliac arteries. The patient was treated by aortobifemoral graft and the ankle and foot ulcers rapidly healed.

Ulceration of mixed arterial and venous origin

Ankle ulceration resulting from a combination of arterial and venous insufficiency is not uncommon, particularly in the elderly. Callam *et al.*[2] found evidence of peripheral arterial insufficiency in 176 (21.3%) of 827 ulcerated legs. It is often not recognised that there is an ischaemic element until months or even years of conventional dressings and compression bandaging fail to achieve satisfactory healing.

History and examination
These patients are more likely to give a history of varicose veins or previous deep vein thrombosis than a history suggestive of arterial insufficiency. Examination is also likely to suggest that the ulcer is purely venous in origin. There is often no obvious cyanosis or other physical sign indicative of a diminished arterial supply. Careful examination of foot pulses is therefore most important in all patients with venous ulceration.

Investigations
Doppler ultrasound examination of ankle pulse pressures is essential, and observation of the toe pulse wave form by PPG may be helpful. Doppler ultrasound is used to identify points of venous incompetence, as in the investigation of uncomplicated venous ulcers. It is often necessary to perform both arteriography and ascending venography to perform full evaluation in order to plan effective treatment in these patients.

Arteriovenous fistulae and venous malformations

Arteriovenous fistulae

These may cause skin ulceration anywhere in the body. Dodd and Cockett describe a patient with ulceration of the shoulder due to a traumatic arteriovenous fistula[3]. Congenital arteriovenous fistulae usually affect the leg (Figure 8.5) and the dilated surface veins may be mistaken for simple varices until their pulsation is noted. Extensive congenital arteriovenous fistulae of one or both limbs, associated with increased blood flow and limb hypertrophy, is known as the Parkes–Weber syndrome.

History
The patient or parents may have been aware of increased limb growth. This is not invariable and superficial venous dilatation is usually thought to be due to simple varicose veins.

Examination
The ulcer is usually indistinguishable in its features from a typical venous ulcer. Careful examination of the surrounding skin will show pulsation of the dilated veins and their bruits can be heard with a stethoscope. Arteriography is necessary to demonstrate the site of the fistula and to evaluate the possibility of therapeutic embolisation.

Traumatic arteriovenous fistulae may be surgically induced. Ulceration of the hand occasionally develops after the formation of a Brescia–Cimino arteriovenous fistula for dialysis in the arm or leg. Arteriovenous fistula formation may also follow inadequate ligation of tributaries of the long saphenous vein when the latter is used for an *in situ* femoropopliteal vein graft. This omission will lead to tender inflammatory induration of the overlying skin, followed by ulceration if the offending tributary is not immediately ligated.

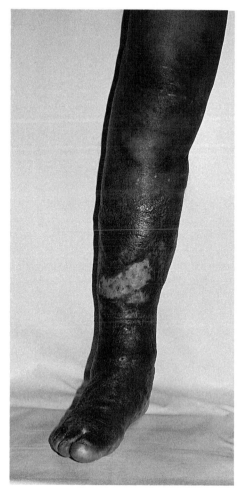

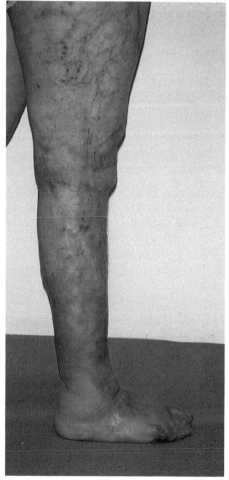

Figure 8.5 Superficial ulceration resulting from congenital arteriovenous fistula

Figure 8.6 Klippel–Trenaunay syndrome; port wine stain on lateral surface of thigh

Venous malformations

The Klippel–Trenaunay syndrome[4] is a congenital disorder, usually affecting one limb only and consisting of a cutaneous naevus ('port-wine stain') on the lateral surface of the thigh, extensive varicose veins, also predominantly on the lateral surface of the thigh, and limb hypertrophy (Figure 8.6). It is distinct from, though often confused with, the Parkes–Weber syndrome. Some patients present with all the features of the Klippel–Trenaunay syndrome apart from limb hypertrophy. This has been described as the 'Klippel-type syndrome'.

Venous ulceration may develop in unusual sites in patients with the Klippel–Trenaunay syndrome or venous haemangiomas.

Case history

A 54-year-old woman presented with a long history of atypical varicose veins, with a capillary haemangioma (port-wine stain) on the lateral surface of the thigh, but without the limb enlargement typical of the true Klippel–Trenaunay syndrome. She had developed extensive ulceration along the posterior surface of the calf. This eventually healed after venographic demonstration of the feeding points of the venous malformation, followed by ligation of these and treatment of the varices by avulsions and injection sclerotherapy.

Contact dermatitis

Contact dermatitis may result in the failure of existing ulcers to heal or in the development of new ulcers. This is usually iatrogenic and due to sensitivity to medicated bandages or local antibiotics. Steroid applications are particularly likely to produce contact dermatitis. The skin is red and scaly and the ulcers are shallow and may appear on any surface of the leg. They are usually not in the malleolar regions. The skin of an ulcer-bearing leg seems to be more sensitive than normal skin and contact dermatitis is a common complication of ulcer dressings. For this reason local antibiotics and medicated dressings and bandages should be scrupulously avoided and replaced by the simple alternatives which are described in Chapter 10.

Rheumatoid and other vasculitic ulcers

If there is a clear history of rheumatoid arthritis, scleroderma, polyarteritis nodosa or other condition with a known tendency to vasculitis, there should be no difficulty in diagnosis. Difficulty does arise when the patient presents with an apparent venous ulcer and without any other obvious manifestations of vasculitis.

Rheumatoid ulcers are usually broad and shallow (Figure 8.7). Frequently multiple, they may affect the lateral or posterior surfaces of the lower leg, but not

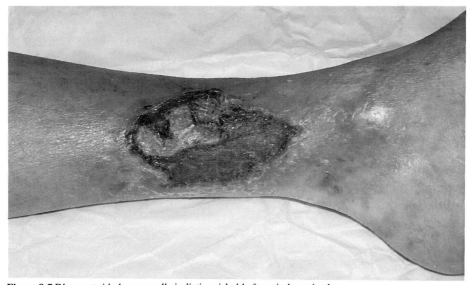

Figure 8.7 Rheumatoid ulcer; usually indistinguishable from ischaemic ulcer

infrequently appear in the malleolar regions and mimic venous ulceration, though usually without surrounding liposclerosis. The base of a rheumatoid ulcer is usually covered by rather pale granulation tissue, often covered by yellow slough, and the edges are poorly epithelialised. A rheumatoid ulcer may look ischaemic but the appearance of ischaemia is usually less marked than ulcers which are secondary to main vessel obstruction. Careful examination of the hands and other joints will usually show evidence of rheumatoid arthritis. The difficult diagnosis is when the ulcer is in malleolar skin and is accompanied by evidence of long or short saphenous incompetence or perforating vein incompetence. If the patient has few or no physical signs of arthritis, a diagnosis of venous ulceration is almost inevitable and, in the author's practice, the rheumatoid component to these ulcers is often overlooked until they fail to respond to conventional venous ulcer treatment.

The other vasculitides usually present with small, often multiple, painful ulcers (Figure 8.8). These may be on the lower leg or foot. Unlike rheumatoid ulcers, they do not normally mimic venous ulceration, and, once it is recognised the ulceration is vasculitic in origin, specific investigations will provide a precise diagnosis.

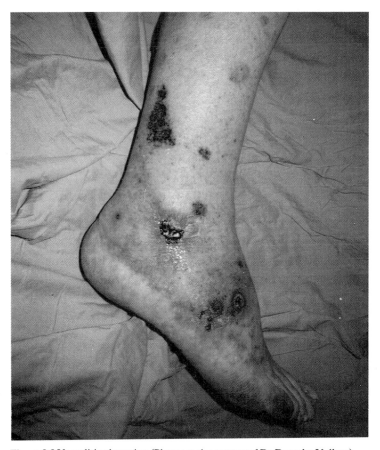

Figure 8.8 Vasculitic ulceration (Photograph courtesy of Dr Dorothy Vollum)

Patients with scleroderma may have the typical tightness of facial skin, resulting in a fixed expression and shiny, tapered fingers. Polyarteritis nodosa may present with a patchy reticular livido on the legs or elsewhere and is often accompanied by muscle tenderness. Systemic lupus erythematosus (SLE) may present with reticulate telangiectatic erythema on the toes and lateral borders of the feet and heels. There may be a butterfly rash across the nose and cheeks. Dilatation of the nail-fold capillaries may occur in either condition. Examination of the veins and of the peripheral pulses is unlikely to show any abnormality.

Investigations

Doppler ultrasound examination is likely to be normal. PPG may demonstrate a damped toe pulse waveform. Specific investigations include the erythrocyte sedimentation rate (ESR) which is likely to be very high. However it must be remembered that a raised ESR may accompany any infected ulcer, whether of venous, arterial or vasculitic origin. Specific investigations for the vasculitides include the Rose–Waaler and latex tests for rheumatoid antibodies and tests for autoantibodies. Antinuclear and DNA antibody titres and DNA binding titres are elevated in lupus erythematosus. Antineutrophil cytoplasmic antibody (ANCA) is elevated in polyarteritis nodosa and in Wegener's granuloma. If scleroderma is suspected, a barium swallow may provide confirmatory evidence; patients with scleroderma typically have uncoordinated oesophageal peristalsis. Smooth muscle incoordination is not necessarily confined to the oesophagus and investigation of a patient in our clinic by barium studies showed normal oesophageal peristalsis; the diagnosis of scleroderma being made by observation of abnormal jejunal peristalsis. In many cases of vasculitis, no specific cause can be identified. If vasculitis is suspected, help in diagnosis and treatment should be sought immediately from a dermatologist or rheumatologist.

Erythrocyanosis

Though not strictly a vasculitis, it is convenient to consider erythrocyanosis here. Erythrocyanosis frigida occurs in young women with fat legs. Areas of skin are mottled and cyanotic and small painful ulcers occasionally occur in these areas. Examination will normally show no arterial or venous disorder and investigations for vasculitis will be negative. These patients may be helped by warm stockings and calcium antagonists and chemical sympathectomy may occasionally be indicated.

Steroid ulcers

Patients undergoing long-term steroid treatment for rheumatoid arthritis, asthma, ulcerative colitis or other conditions are liable to develop ulceration of the leg. These are usually large, shallow, serpiginous ulcers with very poorly epithelialised edges, and the surrounding skin is thin and fragile. They are often similar to rheumatoid ulcers and are notoriously slow to heal. There is usually no difficulty in diagnosis as patients are known to be undergoing steroid therapy. Occasionally a steroid ulcer may mimic a venous ulcer in site and appearance or may co-exist with venous insufficiency. There is then likely to be some confusion in diagnosis.

Case report
A typically difficult case was a 56-year-old diabetic woman with rheumatoid arthritis requiring steroid treatment, with saphenous and perforating vein incompetence and absent foot pulses. Investigation and treatment of each causative lesion was undertaken in turn. The diabetes was controlled as precisely as possible by insulin and diet. Arteriography showed superficial femoral arterial occlusion which was treated by femoropopliteal bypass. The points of venous incompetence were ligated and the steroid therapy was reduced as far as possible. Ulcer healing eventually took place and although there were minor recurrent ulcers in subsequent years, these were smaller than before treatment.

Hypertensive ulcers

Martorell[5] described painful leg ulcers in severely hypertensive patients. Most were situated on the posterior surface of the lower leg, in contrast to typical ischaemic ulcers which are usually on the dorsum of the foot or anterior surface of the leg. It has been suggested that most, if not all, of these ulcers are caused by the embolization of atherosclerotic debris into small skin vessels. However, Martorell described 'hyalinosis' of the tunica intima with stenosis of the arteriolar lumen, and arteriography in Cockett's[6] series of eight patients showed small localized occlusions of the peroneal artery with no obstruction of the posterior tibial or foot arteries.

Diabetic ulcers

Diabetic ulcers may be the result of peripheral neuropathy, ischaemia or infection, or often a combination of all three factors.

Site and appearance
Neuropathic diabetic ulcers are the result of pressure and are therefore usually found on the sole of the foot, commonly under the first metatarsophalangeal joint, or the heel (Figure 8.9). Ischaemic diabetic ulcers may affect the toes or forefoot or the heel, particularly as pressure sores in bed-ridden patients. Diabetic ulcers often result from both ischaemia and neuropathy, with ischaemic slough and surrounding anaesthesia. Less common is necrobiosis lipoidica, ulceration resulting from infection and fat necrosis in the gaiter area of skin of diabetic patients, most of whom are overweight. These ulcers are most likely the result of failure of the skin and subcutaneous tissues of diabetics to respond to minor infection. The infecting organisms are often synergistic, aerobic and microaerophilic organisms combining to cause skin necrosis, as in the synergic ulceration described by Meleney[7].

History
A history of diabetes is usual, but some patients present to an ulcer clinic with previously undiagnosed diabetes. It is therefore essential that urine examination is carried out in all patients. Any patient with glycosuria must be referred immediately to the diabetic clinic for investigation and treatment.

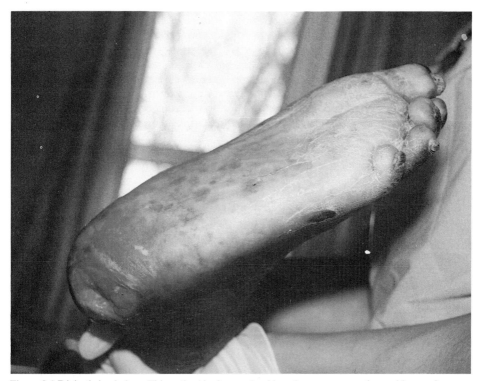

Figure 8.9 Diabetic heel ulcer. This patient had normal ankle pulse pressures and no evidence of proximal atherosclerotic arterial occlusion

Examination
After examining the site and appearance of the ulcers, a neurological examination may show no evidence of peripheral neuropathy. Venous disorders must be excluded by examination and investigations, as has been described, and all leg pulses must be palpated, using Doppler ultrasound examination where necessary.

Investigations
Glycosuria must be further investigated in the diabetic clinic. Absent ankle pulses or reduced pulse pressures must be investigated by arteriography; peripheral ischaemia in diabetes is often attributed solely to small vessel disease and it is important to remember that diabetic patients have a higher than normal incidence of atherosclerosis, which may result in stenosis or occlusion of the main leg vessels. Arteriography may be necessary, even if ankle pressures are apparently within normal limits, as the increased stiffness of diabetic arteries may lead to abnormally high pulse pressures.

Other neuropathies

Patients with paraplegia or peripheral neuropathies may be referred to the ulcer clinic. A diagnosis has usually already been made. However neuropathy may occasionally be diagnosed for the first time in the ulcer clinic. Pressure from poorly fitted calipers may sometimes cause local ulceration. Treatment is usually simple, consisting of healing the ulcer by standard cleaning and dressings followed by appropriate padding to prevent further pressure. Other devices may produce local ischaemia: a young paraplegic patient was recently referred to my clinic with toe ulceration; examination showed that his indwelling urethral catheter was attached to his leg by an excessively tight strap. The ulcer healed when this was removed.

Patients with long-standing peripheral neuropathy may also develop peripheral vascular disorders and these must always be excluded by careful examination and investigations.

Case report
An elderly woman with a long history of muscle wasting due to Charcot–Marie–Tooth disease and with ankle ulceration was found to have absent ankle pulses. Arteriography showed multiple occlusions of the calf arteries.

The message is clear: do not assume that leg or foot ulceration in a patient with peripheral neuropathy is necessarily neuropathic in origin. Always exclude arterial or venous causes by careful examination and investigations.

Traumatic ulceration

Traumatic ulcers may be the result of accidental trauma, self-induced trauma or the result of injection sclerotherapy or operative surgery.

Many patients with venous or ischaemic ulceration give a history of precipitating trauma. Supermarket trolleys have now largely taken over from the steps of buses as causative agents. All patients presenting to an accident and emergency department with abrasions or lacerations of the lower leg should be carefully examined for signs of venous reflux or arterial insufficiency. This is not infrequently overlooked by busy casualty officers and the initial laceration may then develop into chronic ulceration. It should be remembered that abrasions and lacerations of the lower leg and ankle are always slow to heal, particularly in the elderly, even in the presence of normal arteries and veins.

Injection sclerotherapy may cause subcutaneous fat necrosis and ulceration of the overlying skin following extravasation of the sclerosing solution. Sodium tetradecyl sulphate (STD), which is most commonly used for the injection sclerotherapy of varicose veins, is also the most liable to produce painful and indolent ulceration. This not infrequently leads to litigation. Avoidance of such problems is by very careful attention to certain details.

1. Avoid injecting very small varicose veins; extravasation of sclerosant is likely. These are more safely dealt with by avulsion through stab incisions under local anaesthetic.
2. Use a meticulous technique for injection: (a) after inserting the needle into the vein, pull back the syringe plunger and make certain that dark venous blood is aspirated; (b) before injecting the solution, place one finger in front of and another behind the needle so as to localise the injection. Watch the skin over the point of the needle carefully and stop injecting should any swelling appear.

With these simple precautions, ulceration should not occur, or, if it does, it should be sufficiently small to allow simple excision and suture under local anaesthetic.

In injecting venous telangiectasia (spider veins or thread veins), a similarly careful technique should be followed. It is also important to use as non-irritant a solution as possible. STD, diluted three times and shaken into a froth, has been recommended but is very likely to produce unpleasant inflammatory reactions and small ulcers. Sclerovein, a solution of hydroxypolyethoxydodecan in alcohol, is much safer but, in a solution of 1% or greater, may cause small indolent ulcers if there is any extravasation. The 0.5% solution is safer, but often too weak to sclerose the microvarices. Scleremo, a solution of glyceryl chromate, is both effective in sclerosing telangiectasia and also remarkably free of complications.

Factitious ulceration

Traumatic ulcers may be self-induced. It has become a platitude among those who are responsible for ulcer clinics that failure to heal is often the fault of the patient who continually tampers with the ulcer, and it is often said that 'the ulcer is the elderly patient's best friend', intimating that elderly and lonely people may have their only social contact at ulcer clinics or through the district nurse visiting to perform dressings. This attitude is probably an exaggeration of the truth. In the author's series of 77 patients with 109 ulcerated legs, there was one elderly lady whose ulcers mysteriously broke down after a week or two at home, having been perfectly healed after treatment in hospital. She admitted to enjoying the company of others in the ulcer clinic and her chats with doctors and nurses, between which she wrote frequent and very long letters to the surgeon responsible for her treatment. Apart from this lonely woman, the author cannot remember any patient in whom personal interference seemed to be responsible for retarding healing. Factitious ulcers may be quite bizarre in site and appearance, due to being inflicted by such agents as rubber bands tied tightly around the calf. The possibility of self-interference must always be borne in mind in patients whose ulcers are excessively slow in healing, or which recur repeatedly, but the conscientious surgeon will first ask himself whether there is any possible aspect of diagnosis or treatment which could have been overlooked before accusing the patient of self-injury.

Lymphoedema ulcers

Site and appearance
Ulceration is extremely rare in lymphoedema, whether this is primary or secondary to filariasis or malignant involvement of lymph nodes. When they do occur, these ulcers are usually small, indolent and painless and on the anterior surface of the ankle or lower leg.

History
The patient will normally give a long history of swelling of the dorsum of the foot and ankle. The condition is often inherited and primary familial lymphoedema is known as Milroy's disease.

Examination
The limb shows the typical appearances of lymphoedema with marked oedema of the dorsum of the foot. This dorsal foot swelling may sometimes be seen in cardiac

oedema but rarely, if ever, in oedema of purely venous origin. Examination will show no evidence of venous disorder and ankle pulses will normally be present. The oedema may make these difficult to palpate and Doppler ultrasound examination must then be used.

Investigations
Photoplethysmography will distinguish lymphoedema from venous oedema, as described on page 63. Doppler ultrasound examination of ankle pulses is important in any case of doubt and indeed ischaemic ulceration and lymphoedema can co-exist. A patient recently presented to the author's clinic with ulceration in a lymphoedematous leg. Ankle pulses were absent and ankle pulse pressures markedly reduced. The ulcers eventually healed following chemical lumbar sympathectomy. Primary lymphoedema and venous abnormalities can also co-exist, and investigation by Doppler ultrasound examination and venography is then necessary.

The cause of lymphatic insufficiency may be investigated by isotope or X-ray contrast lymphography.

Oedema of other causes

Ulceration may occur in the grossly distended skin of severely oedematous legs in patients with congestive cardiac or renal failure. Examination will usually show no evidence of venous insufficiency, though some impairment of arterial supply is likely to be present in these elderly patients. The ulcers are usually scattered over all surfaces of the leg; they are shallow and may be serpiginous in outline. Treatment must be directed principally at correcting the congestive failure and reducing leg oedema.

Tropical sores and other infections

Tropical sores or ulcers, which are colonised by a variety of pathogenic bacteria, are considered here with other infectious ulcers. This seems appropriate as infectious ulcers of all sorts occur more commonly in tropical and underdeveloped countries than in Northern industrialised societies.

Tropical ulcers

A. D. Landra, a consultant plastic surgeon at Nairobi Hospital[8], defines tropical ulcers as chronic ulcers of the lower leg or dorsum of the foot which occur among the poor populations of tropical countries and are of mixed bacteriology. He excludes those uclers where *Mycobacterium buruli, M. leprae, M. tuberculosis* and Guinea worms have been identified. Anaerobes (fusobacteria) are present in 35% and coliform bacilli in 60% of tropical ulcers. According to Landra, the most common pathogens are *Pseudomonas aeruginosa* and *Proteus mirabilis vulgaris* but MacGraith[9] states that *Treponema vincenti* and *Bacillus fusiformis* are most frequently cultured and can be identified in 80% of smears. The diagnosis of tropical ulcers should exclude ulceration with specific underlying cause such as ischaemia, diabetes or the haemoglobinopathies. Tropical ulcers are more common in males in approximate sex ratio of 2:1. The ulcers are usually single, occasionally multiple, with well-defined raised edges and surrounding oedema. The surface is covered by a greenish-grey foul slough, which pulls away easily to reveal a bleeding granulating base. Predisposing factors are: tropical environment, poverty, malnutrition, chronic anaemia, poor educational standards, lack of hygiene and poor medical facilities. Lack of washing facilities and incentive to keep clean seems to be important; tropical ulceration is less common among Muslim communities in Indonesia, where daily or twice-daily washing is practised, than among similar socioeconomic groups who do not practise this discipline.

Long-standing ulcers may be complicated by periostitis, osteomyelitis or lymphoedema. Malignant change (squamous cell carcinoma) is common in ulcers of between twelve and fifteen years duration, particularly in West Africa and New Guinea.

Other infectious ulcers

Leg ulcers resulting from specific infections are also more common in tropical countries. Tubercular skin ulcers (scrofula) may occur on the legs, but are more common elsewhere. Tuberculous ulcers are characterised by an undermined edge which is irregular, bluish and friable. The ulcers are often multiple and the patient usually has evidence of pulmonary or skeletal tuberculosis. Tuberculous ulceration of the calf has been named erythema induratam scrofulosorum or Bazin's disease. Secondary syphilis has become very rare since the introduction of antibiotics, but occasionally a syphilitic sore may ulcerate, forming a painless, circular punched-out ulcer with a 'wash leather' slough in the base. Yaws may cause similar ulcers.

Other specific infections are leprosy, Guinea worms, caused by the nematode *Dracunculus medinensis*, and anthrax (woolsorter's disease), which rarely occurs on the lower limb. Buruli boil, or Baghdad boil is caused by *Leishmania tropica* and transmitted by a sand fly. Actinomycosis, epidermophytosis, blastomycosis, moniliasis and mycetoma (Madura foot) are other infections which may cause leg ulceration.

Osteomyelitis

Chronic osteomyelitis of the tibia may discharge to form a sinus which may mimic venous ulceration.

Site and appearance
Osteomyelitis may occur anywhere in the leg but is more likely to be mistaken for venous ulceration when it occurs, as commonly happens, in the lower third of the medial surface of the leg. The appearance of necrotic slough is very hard to distinguish from venous ulceration. Osteomyelitis of the toes may occur in association with ischaemic ulceration.

History and examination
There may be a past history of pulmonary or abdominal tuberculosis or a history of local trauma. Examination is unlikely to show any evidence of venous disorder or ischaemia.

Investigations
X-ray examination will normally show bone destruction and sequestrum formation typical of osteomyelitis.

Malignant ulcers

Squamous cell carcinoma

Squamous cell carcinoma developing in an established venous ulcer is known as Marjolin's ulcer[10] (Figure 8.10). Although this complication of venous ulceration is well described in all standard surgical textbooks and is well known to most medical students, it is in fact remarkably rare. Browse *et al.*[11] have reported seeing only five cases in twenty-five years. Ryan and Wilkinson[12] reported only three cases of squamous carcinoma in 2000 ulcers. One or two new cases of leg ulcer are referred

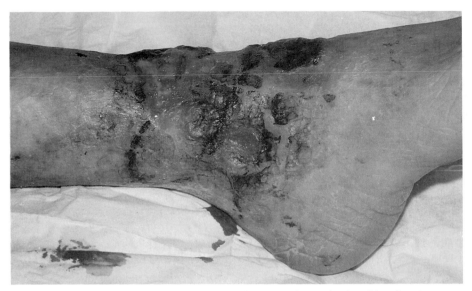

Figure 8.10 Marjolin's ulcer. In this unusual case, squamous carcinoma developed in a chronic venous ulcer following skin grafting. In spite of radiotherapy and below-knee amputation, there was rapid metastatic spread leading to death

to the Lewisham Hospital ulcer clinic each week, a total of between 50 and 100 a year. Only one patient has developed Marjolin's squamous cell carcinoma in a venous ulcer in the past twelve years and the incidence is therefore similar to that reported by Ryan and Wilkinson. This patient's presentation was unusual in that malignant change first developed in the ulcer shortly after treatment by skin grafting. The ulcer had been present for six or seven years, during which time its natural history was similar to that of any other venous ulcer. In spite of radiotherapy followed by below-knee amputation, skin metastases developed in the amputation stump and rapidly spread, cerebral metastases then developed and the patient died within three months of the diagnosis.

Squamous carcinoma should be suspected if there is any overgrowth of tissue in the base or at the edge of the ulcer. Biopsy and histological examination must then be performed as a matter of urgency.

Squamous cell carcinoma may also develop *per primam* on the leg and mimic venous ulceration. In the following case history, a number of alternative diagnoses were considered before the correct one was made.

Case report
A 54-year-old Jamaican woman was referred to the skin clinic with a four-week history of ulceration on the lateral surface of the left ankle. The appearances were typical of an infected venous ulcer (Figure 8.11). She was therefore referred to the vascular clinic where examination and Doppler ultrasound examination failed to show any evidence of venous or arterial disorder. It was then found that she had recently returned from a holiday in Jamaica. She said that she had been walking in the country where there were many thorn bushes and she thought she might have been scratched. It therefore seemed likely that the ulcer was a tropical sore. Biopsy of the ulcer edge showed granulation tissue only, with no evidence of malignancy.

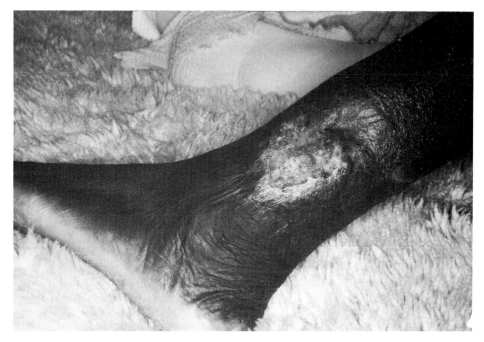

Figure 8.11 Primary squamous carcinoma of the leg. This tumour mimicked a venous ulcer and was diagnosed by biopsy. In spite of below-knee amputation followed by inguinal and iliac block dissection and radiotherapy, the patient died one year after this photograph was taken

X-ray of the leg showed a translucent area in the distal tibia suggestive of osteomyelitis. The diagnosis of tropical sore was abandoned and the patient was referred to an orthopaedic surgeon. The apparent sinus was explored. No osteomyelitis was found but further biopsies of the deep tissues showed that the lesion was in fact a squamous cell carcinoma which had invaded bone. The patient was treated by below-knee amputation. Metastatic spread to the inguinal and iliac lymph nodes occurred eight months later and was treated by block dissection followed by radiotherapy, but in spite of this the patient died after a further four months.

Basal cell carcinoma

Basal cell carcinoma may occasionally occur on the leg. Its appearance is less likely to mimic venous ulceration than squamous cell carcinoma and the diagnosis is established by biopsy. Malignant melanoma is common on the foot and lower leg, but is most unlikely to be confused with venous ulceration.

Sarcomas

Kaposi's sarcoma may present with skin ulceration. The ulcers are usually small and multiple, similar to vasculitic ulcers. Rare at present, ulcerated Kaposi's sarcoma is likely to become an increasing differential diagnosis with the spread of acquired immune deficiency syndrome (AIDS). Tumours of bone, sarcoma and osteoclastoma, may also present with leg ulceration.

Blood dyscrasias

Leg ulceration may occur in conjunction with sickle cell disease, thalassaemia, thrombotic thrombocythaemia, polycythaemia rubra vera and leukaemia. These are usually painful and present as small ischaemic ulcers. In polycythaemia rubra vera, the ischaemia may be sufficient to produce small areas of gangrenous skin on the toes.

Cryoglobulinaemia and macroglobulinaemia cause rouleaux formation of erythrocytes and occlusion of small vessels. This situation is exacerbated by vasospasm and small ischaemic ulcers sometimes result.

Nutritional ulceration

Leg ulceration as a result of malnutrition is most commonly seen in Third World countries accompanying such malnutrition states as kwashiorkor, beriberi and scurvy. The situation is likely to be exacerbated by anaemia, which results from a combination of malnutrition and hook worm infestation.

Leg ulcers were very common among British servicemen in Japanese prisoner-of-war camps during World War II. These 'tropical sores' are likely to have been due to a combination of malnutrition and local trauma resulting in infection. The condition frequently deteriorated into infected gangrene requiring amputation.

It must not be forgotten that malnutrition is not confined to the Third World. The diet of many elderly patients consists mainly of bread and butter, and vitamin C deficiency and anaemia must be considered as possible complicating factors in all elderly patients with venous or ischaemic ulcers. It used to be thought that zinc deficiency was also important and zinc-containing lotions such as lotio rubra were popular in the treatment of leg ulcers. Dietary zinc is mainly obtained from meat, which may be lacking in the diet of elderly patients on low incomes.

Serum zinc levels were measured in over thirty patients attending the St Thomas's Hospital ulcer clinic but no evidence of zinc deficiency was found. Most of these patients were elderly and on low incomes and it was surprising that we were unable to detect any suffering from zinc deficiency. We no longer feel it necessary to check serum zinc levels, except occasionally in elderly patients whose chronic ulcers prove completely resistant to conventional treatment and in whom no other underlying cause can be demonstrated.

Immunodeficiency

Leg ulcers with no evidence of venous ischaemic or other aetiology are now increasingly being seen in HIV-positive Africans[13]. This must obviously be remembered as AIDS becomes more common in the industrialised world.

References

1. Negus, D. Calf pain in the post-thrombotic syndrome. *Br. Med J.* **2**: 156–158, 1968.
2. Callam, M. J., Harper, D. R., Dale, J. J., Ruckley, C. V. Arterial disease in chronic leg ulceration: an underestimated hazard? Lothian and Forth Valley Leg Ulcer Study. *Br. Med. J.* **294**: 929–931, 1987
3. Dodd, H., Cockett, F. B. *The Pathology and Surgery of the Veins of the Lower Limb,* 2nd edn, Edinburgh, Livingstone, p. 254, 1956
4. Klippel, M., Trenaunay, P. Du noevus variqueux osteo-hypertrophique. *Arch. Gen. Med. (Paris)* **185**: 641–672, 1900
5. Martorell, F. Hypertensive ulcer of the leg. *Angiology,* **1**: 133–140, 1950
6. Cockett, F. B. Ulcère de Martorelle. *Phlébologie,* **36**: 363–372, 1983
7. Meleney, F. L. *Clinical Aspects and Treatments of Surgical Infections,* London, Saunders, 1949
8. Landra, A. D. The tropical ulcer. *Surgery* **59**: 1402–1403, 1988
9. MacGraith, B. *Exotic Diseases in Practice,* London, Heinemann, 1965
10. Marjolin, J. N. *Ulcere diet de med (pratique),* Paris, 1846
11. Browse, N. L., Burnand, K. G., Lea Thomas, M. *Diseases of the Veins; Pathology, Diagnosis and Treatment,* London, Arnold, p. 383, 1988
12. Ryan, T. J., Wilkinson, D. S. Diseases of the veins – venous leg ulcers. In *Textbook of Dermatology* (eds Rook, A., Wilkinson, D. S., Ebling, F. J. G.), Oxford, Blackwell Scientific Publications, p. 1098, 1985
13. Bayley, A. C. Surgical pathology of HIV infection: lessons from Africa. *Br. J. Surg.* **77**: 863–867, 1990

Table 8.1 Leg ulcers: a quick guide to diagnosis

Underlying cause	Site	Appearance	Visible veins	Doppler ultrasound	Arteriography	Venography
Varicose	Lower leg, overlying varix	Small, shallow	Large varicose veins	Saphenous incompetence; no ABO	Unnecessary	Unnecessary
Venous (perforating vein ± deep vein incompetence)	Gaiter area of leg, usually medial	Variable size; often infected; healthy granulations when debris removed; usually surrounding liposclerosis	Ankle venous flare; saphenous varicose veins in 50%	ABO; popliteal incompetence in 50%	Unnecessary	ABO ± post-thrombotic deep venous incompetence
Ischaemic	Usually anterior leg, dorsum of foot but may be in gaiter area	Pale base with slough; may be gangrenous areas; poor edge epithelialisation; tendons may be exposed	No varicose veins or venous flare	Reduced ankle pulse pressures	Atherosclerosis: main vessel stenosis on occlusion. Buergers: typical radiological appearance of foot vessels. Vasculitides: normal vessels	Unnecessary
Mixed arterial and venous aetiology	Gaiter area of leg	Indistinguishable from venous ulcer	May be ankle flare and/or varicose veins	May be saphenous incompetence and/or ABO; reduced ankle pulse pressures	Atherosclerotic stenosis or occlusion	May show ABO; deep vein incompetence
Arteriovenous fistula	Over fistula; may be multiple	Usually small; no liposclerosis	May be pulsating varicose veins	Arterial flow audible over fistula	Will demonstrate fistula if sufficiently large	Unnecessary
Klippel–Trenaunay syndrome	Variable, usually related to dilated varices	Typical venous ulcer	Large lateral thigh and extensive leg varices; port-wine stain on lateral thigh	Use to exclude arteriovenous fistula	Unnecessary	May show absent deep veins

Condition	Site	Appearance of ulcer	Associated veins	Ankle pressures	Arteriography	Biopsy
Rheumatoid arthritis	Variable; may mimic venous ulcer	Large, shallow; looks ischaemic; may be multiple	Usually none but may co-exist with varicose veins	Should be normal ankle pulse pressures; if reduced → arteriography	May show multiple stenoses and occlusions	Unnecessary
Other vasculitic ulcers	Variable	Small, multiple	None	Normal	Unnecessary (For specific investigations, see page 97)	Unnecessary
Steroid ulcers	Variable	Large, often multiple; very thin, friable skin	None	Normal	Unnecessary	Unnecessary
Diabetic ulcers	Usually sole of foot or heel	May be 'punched out'; often infected	None	Usually normal or high ankle pulse pressures; if low → arteriography	May show main vessel atherosclerosis	Unnecessary
Lymphoedema (very rare)	Anterior leg	Small, multiple	None	Should be normal, if low, → arteriography (ulcers may be ischaemic)	May show main vessel atherosclerosis	Unnecessary
Tropical sores	Lower leg or foot	Usually single, occasionally multiple; well-defined edges, surrounding oedema, greenish-grey slough in base	None	Normal	Unnecessary	Unnecessary
Marjolin's ulcer	In pre-existing venous ulcer	Ulcer with raised everted edge or nodular irregularity of venous ulcer	May be varicosities or perforating vein incompetence responsible for venous ulcer	As for venous ulcer	Unnecessary	Unnecessary (Diagnosis by biopsy)
Squamous carcinoma	Variable; may be in gaiter area of leg	Raised everted edge or nodular irregularity	None	Normal	Unnecessary	Unnecessary (Diagnosis by biopsy)

ABO, ankle blow-out (Cockett) = perforating vein incompetence.

Chapter 9

Primary ulcer healing

The fundamental principles of healing a leg ulcer apply whether the underlying cause is venous, ischaemic or of other aetiology. Perhaps the most important point which should be made is that the process of ulcer healing is a function of the patient's tissues. There are all too many doctors and nurses under the illusion that they can personally 'heal ulcers', usually by some favourite lotion or dressing. The truth is that the function of the doctor or nurse is simply to counteract those factors which prevent healing so that it can proceed naturally. This means going back to very elementary basic pathology, and remembering that healing is impeded by infection, dependency and oedema, poor blood supply (and in the case of leg ulcers this means venous hypertension at the distal end of the capillary bed as well as inadequate arterial input), diabetes, steroids and trauma.

It is important to provide the most favourable environment for the fibroblasts in the granulation tissue which forms the ulcer base to proliferate so that the ulcer becomes shallower. It is equally important not to interfere with the epithelial growth at the ulcer edge. Leaper and Brennan[1] have performed elegant experiments on cultured fibroblasts and also with the rabbit ear chamber. These have demonstrated that all antiseptics are toxic to fibroblasts, hydrogen peroxide, povidone-iodine and hexachlorophane being the most toxic and chloramine T, a hypochlorite solution, the least toxic in this respect. However hypochlorite solution caused an almost immediate shutdown of the capillaries in the rabbit ear chamber with marked exudation of white and red blood cells. New capillaries did not form for a further ten days. Povidone-iodine (5%) was slightly less toxic to capillaries, with recovery at seventy-two hours. Hydrogen peroxide was innocuous, while chlorhexidine (0.05%) caused a mild exudative reaction and a temporary closing down of a few capillaries only. Leaper concludes that it is better to allow a few bacteria on the surface of a healing ulcer, rather than taking excessive steps to destroy these by strong antiseptics which themselves will inhibit healing. He states that 'hypochlorite solutions may be considered so toxic as to preclude their use in clinical practice in well-defined conditions'. In the author's ulcer clinic, only saline or sterile water is used to clean ulcers. It is even arguable whether the water needs to be sterile; most tap water is sufficiently clean for this purpose.

The infected ulcer

Many ulcers are severely infected when first seen and it is preferable to treat such infection by parenteral antibiotics and to avoid local antiseptics or antibiotics. A swab must be taken for bacteriological examination at the first visit and a two-week course of the appropriate antibiotic is prescribed as soon as the sensitivities are known. Common causative organisms have been described in Chapter 5. *Staphylococcus aureus* is predominant and this is usually sensitive to flucloxacillin. The swabs from the author's clinic were not examined for the presence of anaerobic organisms but Browse *et al.*[2] found anaerobic bacteria in 44% of ulcer cultures. It is obviously advisable therefore to add metronidazole to whatever antibiotic is prescribed for the aerobic organism. Local antibiotic powders should be avoided as allergic reactions are common. Systemically administered antibiotics have been demonstrated to reach the ulcer surface[3]. Scaly skin at the ulcer edge may harbour bacteria and it is wise to clean this away with a little arachis oil, or other light vegetable oil, before cleaning the ulcer itself with water or saline.

Slough in the ulcer base may impede healing and, if not too extensive or thick, this can be removed by various applications. We prefer Debrisan (Pharmacia), a hydrophilic dextranomer, which must be applied twelve-hourly. It is expensive and its prolonged use may inhibit healing. It should be stopped therefore as soon as the slough has been sufficiently removed. Thick eschar or very extensive slough, which particularly occurs in ischaemic ulcers, is best removed surgically. No anaesthetic is usually necessary.

Ulcer cleaning and dressing

As much care should be taken to avoid irritation by dressings as in cleaning. A confusing number of commercial dressings are now available and most nurses and many doctors are confident that the dressing they personally prefer is the only one that should be used. In fact there is little or no scientific evidence that one dressing is better than another. The important principle is that any dressing should be non-irritant and that exudate from the ulcer surface should be absorbed. Blair and his colleagues[4] demonstrated that 74% of venous ulcers healed completely within twelve weeks with regular cleaning, dressings and sustained compression (four-layer) bandaging. They did not report any difference in effectiveness between non-adherent dry dressing (N-A Dressing; sterile knitted viscose primary dressing), Granuflex (occlusive dressings) and Flamazine (antibiotic impregnated dressings).

The long-established medicated dressings, Calaband and Ichthopaste, are still in common use but are liable to produce allergic reactions. More modern absorbent and occlusive dressings such as Scherisorb (Schering), Sorbsan (NI Medical) and Granuflex (Squibb Surgical) are less liable to produce side-effects and, apart from their expense, there is no particular objection to these. Melolin (Smith & Nephew) should be avoided as its poor absorbent properties make it liable to produce skin maceration. Plain cotton gauze is absorbent and unlikely to produce any allergic reaction (though this has been described). The problem with gauze is that it adheres to the surface of the ulcer and is painful to remove. Paraffin gauze dressings such as Jelonet (Smith & Nephew), Paratulle (Seton) and Coban (3M) have excellent non-adherent properties and are easy to apply and remove, but also have the disadvantage of occasionally giving rise to allergic reactions. Most local applications, particularly steroids and zinc powder or lotion, may also produce allergic dermatitis.

The standard regimen in the author's clinic is to clean the ulcer with sterile water or saline after removing scurfy surrounding skin with light vegetable oil and then to apply N-A Dressing (Johnson & Johnson) (Figure 9.1). This is covered by

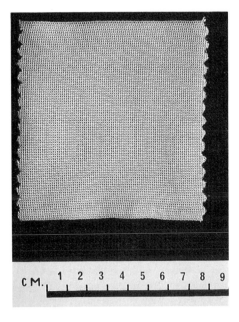

Figure 9.1 Non-adhesive dry dressing (N-A Dressing) (sterile knitted viscose primary dressing, BP, Johnson and Johnson)

absorbent cotton gauze and then the leg is bandaged; firmly if the ulcer is venous in origin but lightly if it is ishaemic. N-A Dressing is sterile knitted viscose primary dressing, and Tricotex (Smith & Nephew) is very similar. These dressings have the advantage of having very large pores which allow exudate to pass through them. They are not in themselves absorbent and must therefore be backed up by absorbent cotton gauze.

In using the combination of a non-adherent sterile knitted viscose primary dressing (N-A Dressing or Tricotex) and gauze dressings it is most important to ensure that the gauze is made of cotton and not the (much less absorbent) paper 'gauze' which is too often supplied to ulcer clinics in NHS hospitals in the interests of economy.

Compression bandaging

Venous ulcers require firm compression to counteract venous hypertension and effect healing. A number of bandages and stockings are available and there is some division of opinion as to whether bandages or stockings should be used. The advantage of using medium compression elastic stockings is that they maintain their compression considerably better than bandages and, as their durability is greater than that of bandages, their is little difference in overall expense. The main disadvantage of stockings is their liability to soiling from exudate and it is easier and less expensive to apply a second bandage while the first is washed than to prescribe several pairs of stockings. The other disadvantage of elastic stockings is that they may be difficult for the patient to apply at home and many of the author's patients undertake their own ulcer dressing and cleaning, usually with the help of a relative or friend.

The main disadvantage of bandaging is the very poor standards achieved by modern doctors and nurses. Mrs Dale, a senior community nurse from Edinburgh[5], found that nurses trained locally only receive one hour of instruction in bandaging during their whole three-year training programme and the situation is probably no different in most nursing schools. Firm compression is essential to achieve successful ulcer healing and this is simply not applied by inexperienced nurses or doctors.

In the Lewisham ulcer clinic we use a medium-weight elasticated bandage (Elastocrepe; Smith & Nephew) and this is then covered by Tubigrip tubular gauze (Seton). The purpose of the 'tube-gauze' is both slightly to increase the degree of compression and to prevent the bandage slipping and losing its compression, as has been demonstrated by Mrs Dale and her colleagues. We have not performed detailed studies of this method, but patients find the combination of Elastocrepe and Tubigrip comfortable and most have no difficulty in applying these themselves.

Stronger bandages which are available include the Bisgaard bandage, Coban (which is self-adhesive and therefore prevented from slipping), the Dixon-Wright bandage and the Elastoweb bandage. The heavier bandages should be available in a clinic and are useful for the patient with very severe oedema or very large legs. Moffat and his colleagues[6] have achieved a 92% healing rate of venous ulcers in a mean twelve weeks with the use of high compression (four-layer) bandaging.

Bandaging techniques

Mrs Dale has made a teaching video recording which demonstrates bandaging techniques[7]. Millard and his colleagues[8], using the Borgnis medical stocking tester, demonstrated a range of stocking pressures at the ankle from 5 to 51 mmHg following application by untrained nurses. Four of the nine nurses applied the bandages at less than 15 mmHg at the ankle, which is not regarded as an adequate pressure. Following instruction, all nurses achieved pressures at the ankle of greater than 15 mmHg and most obtained adequate graduation of pressure up the leg.

The essential features of compression bandaging in the treatment of leg ulceration are:

1. Adequate pressure (more than 15 mmHg at the ankle).
2. Graduated compression from ankle to knee.

This may be achieved by the following technique (Figure 9.2). The bandage is first locked around the forefoot by an overlapping turn. The bandage is then wound up over the ankle and the heel is covered. Bandaging continues up the leg by single overlapping turns, each turn covering half the width of the previous turn. The bandage is extended fully as it is applied and then allowed to relax to about 70% of its full stretched length. It is most important to include the heel in the bandage; omission will result in a tourniquet affect at the ankle and oedema of the foot. As mentioned above, we then apply size D or E Tubigrip over the bandage to prevent slippage and to help maintain compression. Alternatively a self-adhesive bandage (Coband or Lohmann) may be used. It is advisable for doctors and nurses working in an ulcer clinic to check that they are achieving adequate ankle pressures and graduation up the leg by using a Borgnis medical stocking pressure tester on their first two or three patients and to recheck their performance until this is consistently satisfactory.

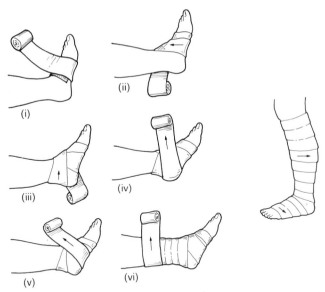

(i)

(ii)

(iii)

(iv)

(v)

(vi)

Figure 9.2 The standard bandaging technique. Two important points: (1) enclose the heel; (2) each turn overlaps the previous turn by half its width

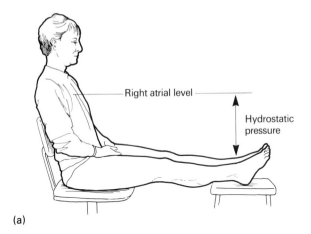

Right atrial level

Hydrostatic pressure

(a)

Right atrial level

(b)

Figure 9.3 Leg elevation: (a) the wrong, and (b) the right way

Elevation

Patients being treated for venous ulceration by dressings and compression bandaging must be firmly advised to avoid prolonged standing and to rest with the leg well elevated as much as possible. Simply elevating the leg on a stool or chair (Figure 9.3a) while sitting upright is both uncomfortable and ineffectual. The leg must be elevated to heart level by lying back on a sofa or bed so that the foot and ankle are at or above the level of the right atrium. The best designed piece of furniture for this purpose is a garden lounger (Figure 9.3b). Patients' and nurses' co-operation can easily be achieved by a simple description of the hydrostatic pressures involved in venous return to the heart.

Elevation and dressings can usually be carried out in the patient's home; admission to hospital is only necessary for the most severe ulcers or in unacceptable social conditions.

Skin grafting

Most venous uclers, 80% in the Lewisham series, heal in a mean three months with dressings and firm compression bandaging. Only a minority therefore require skin grafting, but the numbers may be significant in a large ulcer clinic. Venous ulcers can be grafted either after ligation of incompetent perforating and saphenous veins, with excision of the ulcer bed, or at the same time as the venous surgery is undertaken. We prefer the latter approach, as it reduces operating time and, with appropriate antibiotic cover, there have been no problems of wound infection. However, it is probably wiser to treat the grossly infected long-standing chronic ulcer by Cockett's technique of delayed grafting following surgical excision of the grossly infected tissues.

Ischaemic ulcers usually require grafting but it is essential to relieve the ischaemia as far as possible, by the methods described in Chapter 11, before any attempt to graft is made. A chronically infected ischaemic ulcer in a patient requiring arterial reconstruction, particularly where synthetic grafts may be necessary, should be treated similarly to Cockett's method of treating venous ulcers. Following ten days appropriate antibiotic therapy, the ulcer is excised under general anaesthetic, antibiotics are continued and the arterial graft is performed two or three days later. Skin grafting can be performed under the same anaesthetic or later, if any doubt is felt about the success of revascularising the ulcer bed.

Split skin or pinch grafts?
Split skin grafts taken from the ipsilateral thigh are quick and easy to perform, using either a Humby knife or an electric dermatome. The graft must be thoroughly perforated, to allow for the release of exudate which might otherwise lift it from the underlying tissues, and is sutured in place using interrupted 2–0 black silk sutures. One end of each suture is left long. The graft is covered with tulle gras dressing and this by a flavine wool pack. This ingenious dressing, invented by the late Mr 'Dickie' Battle of St Thomas's Hospital, consists of a lump of cotton wool thoroughly soaked in flavine emulsion and kneaded until it attains a doughy consistency. This is placed over the graft dressing and is held in place by tying together the long ends of the sutures round the graft edge. The whole is covered by more dressing gauze followed by a crepe bandage. A plaster of Paris back slab may be indicated if it is felt likely that the patient will move his ankle while the graft is

taking. This is usually not necessary in patients with venous ulcers as they often have severely limited ankle movements.

A more satisfactory method, in the author's view, is to use pinch grafts. These are taken either from the lower abdominal wall or from the ipsilateral thigh. If only a small ulcer requires cover, it is kind to the patient to remove the grafts in a line after infiltration with a local anaesthetic. The intervening skin can then be excised and the line sutured to form a linear wound. This is a great deal less painful than the donor areas resulting from split skin grafting or extensive pinch grafts. Following infiltration of local anaesthetic, small roundels of skin about 1 cm in diameter are excised by lifting the centre of each, either by a needle or by using fine-toothed forceps, e.g. Adson's. The roundel of skin is then excised using a large-bladed scalpel knife; the author finds a Gillette A blade most suitable for this. Care must be taken to remove any fat from the undersurface of each roundel. These are then

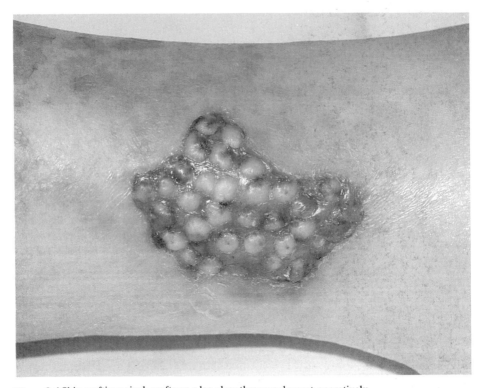

Figure 9.4 Skin grafting: pinch grafts on a leg ulcer three weeks post-operatively

placed on the ulcer bed (Figure 9.4), gaps of 2–3 mm being left between each to allow for their expansion when pressure is applied. The grafts are covered with tulle gras and a flavine pack and bandaged, as has been described for split skin grafts.

Pinch grafting includes small areas of dermis in each graft and the finished product is stronger than that resulting from split skin grafting. If a very large ulcer has to be grafted however, it may be felt that the extent of the donor site is unacceptable and split skin grafting may then be preferred.

Cross-leg flap grafting or vascularised free flap grafts have been described but this author has no experience of these. The most intractable ulcers are the result of persistent underlying venous hypertension or ischaemia and more attention should be paid to correcting the underlying abnormality than to new approaches to skin cover. For example, Browse et al.[9] describe a patient who underwent a cross-leg flap for persistent venous ulceration lasting for more than fifteen years following communicating vein ligation, deep venous reconstruction and the continuous use of graduated elastic stockings. Healing was initially successful but the grafted area developed lipodermatosclerosis two years later and this subsequently ulcerated. We also have experience of patients whose ulcers became completely intractable, usually due to a combination of very severe underlying venous disorder and some degree of ischaemia.

Pharmacological treatment of leg ulcers

Although many claims have been made by pharmaceutical companies, the pharmacological treatment of venous disorders, including ulceration, is still in its very early stages. Encouraging results have been achieved in healing ischaemic ulcers by the use of the vasoactive prostaglandins, PGE_1 and PGI_2 (prostacyclin), but the place of drugs in the treatment of venous ulceration is less certain.

Venoactive drugs in the treatment of venous ulceration

This subheading should be followed by the words 'Watch this space'. At present, drugs may have some marginal effect in the healing of venous ulcers but, with the possible exception of stanozolol and oxpentifylline, there is no evidence that any of the presently available drugs is as effective as mechanical methods in the treatment of venous ulceration. Those involved in the management of venous ulcers should however be aware of the possibility of future developments in pharmacological products and be sufficiently open-minded to try these if their developments are supported by carefully conducted clinical trials.

There are now a number of hypotheses about the microcirculatory changes which underlie lipodermatosclerosis and ulceration and these are described in Chapter 5. Each of the drugs listed below is aimed at counteracting one or more of the microcirculatory abnormalities and these are indicated in each subheading.

At the present time there are five drugs with some claim to usefulness in the management of venous disorders.

Stanozolol (fibrinolytic enhancement)
Stanozolol (Stromba; Sterling-Winthrop) has a long-term effect in stimulating natural fibrinolysis[10]. Browse et al. and Burnand et al. have demonstrated its usefulness in the treatment of lipodermatosclerosis in a pilot study[11] and a double-blind cross-over trial[12]. Significant decrease in the area of lipodermatosclerosis was accompanied by a demonstrable increase in fibrinolytic activity and a significant fall in plasma fibrinogen. The usual dose is 10 mg b.d., though some patients cannot tolerate this due to nausea.

There is no doubt that stanozolol is a most helpful drug in the treatment of patients with painful inflammatory lipodermatosclerosis. Its effect on the long-term healing of venous ulcers is less clear. Burnand and his colleagues[13] have reported a controlled trial in which half their patients were treated by stanozolol for nine months and the other half underwent surgery to eradicate all sites of superficial valvular incompetence. Both groups wore elastic stockings continuously during and after the treatment. There was no difference in the numbers of patients developing further ulceration within four years of entry into the trial. They conclude that stanozolol and stockings appear to be as efficacious as surgery and stockings in preventing the recurrence of venous ulceration. They do not indicate how many patients in each group had deep venous incompetence and how many had only perforating vein and superficial venous incompetence. As Burnand and his colleagues[14] had previously shown that perforating vein ligation in patients without deep venous damage is followed by satisfactory long-term results, it would seem unnecessary that such patients should have to wear elastic compression stockings for the rest of their lives.

The disadvantage of stanozolol is that it is slow to produce beneficial effects; the drug usually has to be taken for about six weeks before any benefit is demonstrable, and it may also cause nausea and, through its mildly androgenic action, virilising effects, oligomenorrhoea, acne and very rarely hirsutism; it is contraindicated in premenopausal women. These side-effects are sufficient to prevent continued treatment in a significant number of patients, and the manufacturers no longer recommend it for the treatment of liposclerosis or venous ulceration.

Defibrotide (fibrinolytic enhancement)
Belcaro and Marelli[15] have investigated the effects of defibrotide (Roussel–Maestretti, Milan), a profibrinolytic and antithrombotic drug, in patients with venous hypertension, lipodermatosclerosis and ulceration in a controlled trial. No side-effects were observed. Combined treatment by defibrotide and elastic compression was significantly more effective in reducing both liposclerosis and ulceration and in improving microcirculatory parameters and capillary permeability.

Oxpentifylline (inhibition of leucocyte aggregation + ? fibrinolytic enhancement)
Originally developed for the treatment of ischaemia, oxpentifylline (Trental; Hoechst) has been demonstrated to inhibit granulocyte aggregation and the production of oxidants from granulocytes. This appears to have a protective effect on erythrocytes, whose filterability is altered by leukotriene B_4[16]. It has also been suggested that leucocytes elaborate either tissue-type plasminogen activator or urokinase and that, through this mechanism, oxpentifylline can increase the rate of fibrinolysis. Oral and parenteral administration of oxpentifylline to patients with peripheral vascular disease has led to decreased fibrinogen levels, either due to increased fibrinolytic activity or to a reduction of fibrinogen production[17]. Marked improvement in ischaemic ulceration has been demonstrated in between 60 and 87% of patients treated with 400 mg/day or more[18-20]. Beneficial effects in leg ulcers secondary to thalassaemia have been reported in a small study[21].

In a small and uncontrolled study of ten patients whose leg ulcers were considered to be due to a combination of deep venous incompetence and moderate ischaemia, Angelides *et al.* considered that oxpentifylline had a beneficial effect on ulcer healing[22]. A multicentre study in four centres in England and Ireland[23] investigated the efficacy of oxpentifylline in the treatment of venous ulceration. Patients with peripheral arterial disease were excluded and 80 patients were randomised to receive oxpentifylline 400 mg three times daily or placebo, in addition to optimum conservative therapy (the nature of which is not explained). Treatment was continued for six months or until the index ulcer healed, if this occurred sooner. Complete healing occurred in 35 patients (oxpentifylline 23, placebo 12) and the authors conclude from these results that oxpentifylline may be a useful drug in the treatment of venous ulceration.

Vasoactive prostaglandins (vasodilator and inhibition of platelet adhesiveness)
The vasoactive prostaglandins, PGE_1 and PGI_2 (prostacyclin, epoprostenol, Flolan; Wellcome) are powerful vasodilators and inhibit platelet aggregation. Intravenous prostacyclin in glycine buffer was compared to the placebo effect of glycine buffer alone in a randomised study of 30 patients with 52 ischaemic leg ulcers by Nizankowski and his colleagues in 1985[24]. A significant reduction in ulcer size in patients receiving prostacyclin was accompanied by reduction in rest pain. The role of prostaglandins in the treatment of venous ucleration has only recently been investigated. Rudofsky and Hajek[25] reported a double-blind placebo-controlled trial of intravenous PGE_1 in the treatment of venous ulcers. They concluded that PGE_1 treatment, compared to placebo, resulted in a significantly ($P < 0.001$) better reduction or healing of ulcers accompanied by improvement in venous haemodynamic parameters. In a small study of 10 patients with severe skin ischaemia in progressive systemic sclerosis, treated by intravenous infusion of the PGI_2 analogue, Iloprost, Guilmot and his colleagues[26] reported pain relief in 9 of 10 patients and healing of ulcers in 2 of 3 patients. This is an uncontrolled pilot study, but its results should encourage further investigation by a controlled trial.

Venoruton (improvement of microvascular permeability)
Venoruton, O-(β-hydroxyethyl)-rotoside (HR) (Paroven; Zyma), is a semi-synthetic flavinoid. HR is a standardised mixture of monohydroxyethylrutosides (5–10%), dihydroxyethylrutosides (30–38%), trihydroxyethylrutosides (45–55%) and tetrahydroxyethylrutosides (3–12%). These compounds have been demons-trated to inhibit microvascular permeability and oedema formation[27]. Michel et al.[28] demonstrated a decrease in permeability of single perfused capillaries and venules in the frog mesentery resulting from the effect of hydroxyethylrutosides. Further identification and concentration of the most active ingredients might improve its clinical efficacy[29].

The efficacy of the hydroxyrutosides in the treatment of venous ulceration is less well documented. Neumann and Van de Broek have demonstrated a significant increase in $TcPo_2$ in patients with chronic venous insufficiency treated by HR[30] and Diebschlag et al. demonstrated a dose-related reduction in leg volume in patients with chronic insufficiency[31]. Patients treated by a combination of venoruton (Paroven) and elastic stockings have shown a lower rate of venous ulcer recurrence than those treated by placebo and elastic support treatment[32]. In a second trial[33], it was demonstrated that ulcer surface area decreased to a markedly greater extent following venoruton plus compression treatment, compared to compression therapy alone.

Other pharmacological agents under investigation for the treatment of venous ulceration and other disorders

Urokinase (fibrinolysis)
Microthrombi in the vicinity of leg ulcers have been demonstrated by a number of authors[34] and Ehrly and his colleagues[35] have investigated the effect of low-dose,

long-term urokinase therapy in patients with venous leg ulcers. This was only a small uncontrolled study, but the authors did demonstrate a continuous and significant increase in $TcPo_2$ values over a four-week period. Mean ulcer area reduced from $19.05\,cm^2$ to $5.27\,cm^2$. The results of this study are open to criticism; apart from the small number of patients and lack of controls, all patients were in hospital during treatment and were being treated 'with ointment, compression and so on'. A larger controlled study will have to be undertaken before any conclusions can be made about the possible place of urokinase in healing venous ulcers.

Diosmine-flavinoids (capillary permeability)
Cospite and his colleagues[36] have demonstrated a reduction in the capillary filtration curve coefficient and thus the capillary permeability by the administration of diosmine-flavinoids to patients with primary varicose veins and perforating vein incompetence. There is no mention of their use in the treatment of venous ulceration.

Venostasin retard (inhibition of leg oedema)
Venostasin retard is an extract of horse chestnut seed. A small controlled study[37] of nineteen subjects on a fifteen hour flight from London to Tokyo demonstrated that those receiving Venostasin developed significantly less leg swelling than subjects receiving placebo. No studies of the effect of this drug on venous ulceration have yet been carried out.

Summary

Of the many drugs which have recently been developed and which have been described here, stanozolol (Stromba) and oxpentifylline (Trental) are both supported by a number of well-conducted clinical studies. Even these drugs can play only a small part in ulcer management, but they may be of use as adjuvants in initial ulcer healing and also for longer-term therapy in patients unfit for surgery or in those where surgery is ineffectual.

Stanozolol is of proven value in the treatment of lipodermatosclerosis but its place in the management of venous ulceration is more controversial, particularly in view of its troublesome side-effects. The principal use of oxpentifylline is in the treatment of ischaemia and it is likely to be most useful in treating ulcers of mixed arterial and venous aetiology or where the ulcer is thought to be primarily venous in origin but some of ischaemia is suspected.

References

1. Leaper, D. J., Brennan, S. S. Let's have a rethink about the use of antiseptics for venous ulcers. In *Phlebology '85* (eds Negus, D., Jantet, G.), London, Libbey, pp. 580–583, 1986
2. Browse, N. L., Burnand, K. G., Lea Thomas, M. *Diseases of the Veins; Pathology, Diagnosis and Treatment,* London, Arnold, p. 406, 1988
3. Hopkins, N. F. G., Jamieson, C. W. Antibiotic concentration in exudate in venous ulcers; the prediction of ulcer healing rate. *Br. J. Surg.* **70**: 532–534, 1983
4. Blair, S. D., Wright, D. D. I., Backhouse, C. M., Riddle, E., McCallum, C. N. Sustained compression and healing of chronic venous ulcers. *Br. Med. J.* **297**: 1159–1161, 1988
5. Dale, J. Callam, M., Ruckley, C. V. How efficient is a compressive bandage? *Nurs. Times* **79**: 46, 49–51, 1983

6. Moffat, C., Wright, D. D. I., Franks, P. J., Oldroyd, N., Greenhalgh, R. N., McCallum, C. N. Healing chronic venous ulcers: a community problem. In *Phlebology '89* (eds Davey, A., Stemmer, R.), Paris, Libbey, pp. 1139–1141, 1989

7. Dale, J. J., Callum, M. J., Gibson, B., Harper, D. R., Ruckley, C. V. Bandaging for leg ulcers. A video recording for teaching health care workers and patients. In *Phlebology '85* (eds Negus, D., Jantet, G.), London, Libbey, pp. 643–645, 1986

8. Millard, L. G., Bleacher, A., Fentem, P. H. The pressure at which nursing staff apply compression bandages when treating patients with varicose ulcers. In *Phlebology '85* (eds Negus, D., Jantet, G.), London, Libbey, pp. 682–685, 1986

9. Browse, N. L., Burnand, K. G., Lea Thomas, M. *Diseases of the Veins; Pathology, Diagnosis and Treatment*, London, Arnold, pp. 427–428, 1988

10. Davidson, J. F., Lockhead, N., McDonald, G. A., McNicol, G. P. Fibrinolytic enhancement by stanozolol. A double-blind trail. *Br. J. Haematol.* **22**: 543–559, 1972

11. Browse, N. L., Jarrett, P. E. M., Morland, M., Burnand, K. G. The treatment of liposclerosis of the leg by fibrinolytic enhancement: a preliminary report. *Br. Med. J.* **7**: 434–435, 1977

12. Burnand, K. G., Clemenson, G., Morland, M., Jarrett, P. E. M., Brose, N. L. Venous lipodermatosclerosis, treatment by fibrinolytic enhancement and elastic compression. *Br. Med. J.* **280**: 7, 1980

13. Burnand, K. G., Stacey, M. C., Blair, G. T., Lloyd, K., De Beaux, F., Browse, N. L. Fibrinolytic enhancement versus surgical ablation of superficial incompetence in the prevention of venous ulcer recurrence: a controlled clinical trial. *Br. J. Surg.* **76**: 418, 1989

14. Burnand, K. G., Lea Thomas, M., O'Donnell, T., Browse, N. L. The relationship between post-phlebitic changes in the deep veins and results of surgical treatment of venous ulcers. *Lancet* **2**: 936–938, 1976

15. Belcaro, G., Marelli, C. Treatment of venous lipodermatosclerosis and ulceration in venous hypertension by elastic compression and fibrinolytic enhancement with defibrotide. *Phlebology* **4**: 91–106, 1989

16. Freyburger. G., Hammerschmidt, D. E., Coppo, P. A., Baisscou, M. R. Leucocyte activation and rheological changes: effect of pentoxifylline. In *Pentoxifylline and Leucocyte Function* (eds Mondal, G. L., Novick, W. J.), Sommerville, New Jersey, Hoechst-Roussel Pharmaceuticals, p. 82, 1988

17. Jarrett, P. E. M., Marland, M., Browse, N. L. The effect of oxpentifylline on fibrinolytic activity and plasma fibrinogen levels. *Curr. Med. Res. Opin.* **4**: 492–495, 1977

18. Bosson, G. W. Klinische Erfahrungen mit dem Vasotherapeutikum Trental in der Dermatologie. *Z. Hautkr.* **46**: 711–724, 1972

19. Herger, R. Erfahrungen mit dem neuen Vasotherapeutikum Trental in der dermatologischen Fachpraxis. *Fortschr. Med.* **24**: 865–872, 1972

20. Weitgasscer, H. The use of pentoxifylline (Trental 400) in the treatment of leg ulcers: results of a double-blind trail. *Pharmatherapeutica* **3** (suppl. 1): 143–151, 1983

21. Forteleoni, G., Pacitti, C., Mulas, G., *et al.* La nostra esperienza nel trattamento delle ulcere malleolari nella talessemia. *Terapia* **74**: 1173–1178, 1983

22. Angelides, N. S., von der Ahe, W. Effect of oral pentoxifylline on leg ulcers due to deep venous incompetence in patients with a concomitant moderate arterial disease. In *Phlébologie '89* (eds Davy, A., Stemmer, R.), Paris. Libbey, p. 1145, 1989

23. Colgan, M-P., Dormandy, J., Jones, P., Shannik, G., Schraibman, I., Young, R. The efficacy of Trental in the treatment of venous ulceration. In *Phlébologie '89* (eds Davy, A., Stemmer, R.), Paris, Libbey, p. 1154, 1989

24. Nizankowski, R., Krolikowski, W., Bielatowicz, J., Schaller, J., Szceklik, A. Prostacyclin for ischemic ulcers in peripheral arterial disease: a random assignment, placebo-controlled study. In *Prostacyclin – Clinical Trials* (eds Gryglewski, R. J., Szceklik, A., McCiff, J. C.), New York, Raven Press, p. 15, 1985

25. Rudofsky, G., Hajek, B. Intravenous prostacyclin E_1 in the treatment of venous ulcers – a double-blind, placebo-controlled trial. *Abstracts of the 15th World Congress, International Union of Angiology*, Rome, September, p. 425, 1989

26. Guilmot, J. L., Lasfargues, G., Diot, E., *et al.* Severe skin ischaemia in progressive systemic sclerosis; treatment with PGI_2 analog (Iloprost) in 10 patients. *Abstracts of the 15th World Congress, International Union of Angiology,* Rome, September, p. 211, 1989

27. Artuson, G. Effects of O-(β-hydroxyethyl)-rutosides (HR) on the increased microvascular permeability in experimental skin burns. *Acta Chir. Scan.* **138**: 111–117, 1972
28. Michel, C., Blumberg, S., Clough, G. Hydroxyethyl-rutosides (HR) reduce permeability of frog mesenteric microvessels. *Phlebology.* **5** (Suppl. 1), 3–7, 1990
29. Michel, C. Personal communication, 1989
30. Neumann, H. A. M., van den Broek, J. J. T. B. Evaluation of O-(β-hydroxyethyl)-rutosides in chronic venous insufficiency by means of non-invasive techniques. *Phlebology.* **5** (Suppl. 1), 13–20, 1990
31. Nocker, W., Diebschlag, W., Lemmacher, W. Clinical trails of the dose-related effects of O-(β-hydroxyethyl)-rutosides in patients with chronic venous insufficiency. *Phlebology.* **5** (Suppl. 1), 23–26, 1990
32. Ruckley, C. V., Neumann, H. A. M., Krumberg, N. H. D. *et al.*, Prevention of breakdown of venous ulcer with Venorouton O-(β-hydroxyethyl-rutosides, HR). A long-term placebo-controlled trial. *Abstracts of the Congress of the International Union of Phlebology,* Essen, November, 1987
33. Stegmann, W., Huebner, K., Deichmann, B., Mueller, B., Wirksamkeit, der O. O-(β-hydroxyethyl)-rutoside bei der Behandlung des venösen Ulcus cruris. *Therapiewoche* **36**: 1828–1833, 1986
34. Ehrly, A. M., Partsch, H. Microcirculatory and haemorrheologic abnormalities in venous leg ulcers: introductory remarks. In *Phlébologie '89* (eds Davy, A., Stemmer, R.), Paris, Libbey, p. 142, 1989
35. Ehrly, A. M., Schenk, J., Bromberger, U. Effects of low dose, long-term urokinase on TcPo₂ of patients with venous leg ulcers. In *Phlébologie 89* (eds Davy, A., Stemmer, R.), Paris, Libbey, p. 147, 1989
36. Cospite, M., Ferrara, F., Milio, G., Scrivano, V., Meli, F., Lo Presti, T. Diosmine-flavinoids and microcirculation in venous disease of lower limbs. *Abstracts of the 15th World Congress, International Union of Angiology,* Rome, September, p. 116, 1989
37. Marshall, M., Dormandy, J. A. Oedema of long distance flights. *Phlebology* **2**: 123–124, 1987

Chapter 10

Definitive treatment: prevention of recurrence of venous ulceration

Too many doctors and nurses feel that they have done all they can for the patient in their care when they have succeeded in healing a venous ulcer by dressings and compression bandaging. This is only half the story. In the Lewisham Hospital series of 77 patients with 109 ulcerated legs, patients presenting to the clinic gave histories of recurrent ulceration ranging from a few months to over 50 years, with a mean of 16.6 years[1]. All had been treated previously by dressings and compression bandaging and some also by injection sclerotherapy or by ligation and stripping of incompetent saphenous veins. The Lothian and Forth Valley Ulcer Study provides an equally gloomy commentary on the conservative treatment of venous ulceration; of these patients, 45% had suffered from intermittent ulceration for more than 10 years[2]. Cornwall *et al.* found a 46% ulcer recurrence rate in 109 patients treated conservatively, by compression stockings, after initial ulcer healing[3]. These figures indicate the inadequacy of compression stockings alone in preventing recurrent venous ulceration.

This chapter describes control of the various sites of venous incompetence by injection sclerotherapy or surgery in order to prevent recurrent ulceration. There are, in addition, a number of pharmacological agents which have been described in Chapter 9. At present their development is insufficiently advanced to take over the role of the surgeon, but doubtless further developments will take place in this field and those responsible for ulcer clinics, whether surgeons or dermatologists, should keep a careful eye on the literature and, where any pharmacological agent is shown effective by clinical trial, this should be included in the treatment plan.

Varicose veins

As has been emphasized, varicose ulceration, that is ulceration as the result of long or short saphenous incompetence, without deep vein or perforating vein incompetence, is rare. It is however appropriate to discuss the surgery of long and short saphenous veins as these often require treatment in the management of venous ulceration.

Before performing injection sclerotherapy or surgery, the ulcer should be healed if possible. As varicose ulcers are normally small and shallow this should present no difficulty; dressings and compression bandages usually effect complete healing within a few weeks.

Superficial varicose veins can be treated either by injection sclerotherapy or by surgery. Hobbs[4] has shown that the results of injection sclerotherapy are very poor indeed in the presence of long or short saphenous incompetence, with an 80% recurrence rate, and the results of treating thigh varices are also poor. Injection sclerotherapy is therefore best reserved for isolated varices, without demonstrable long or short saphenous incompetence, in the calf or knee region. Hobbs also recommends treating incompetent calf perforating veins by injection sclerotherapy, but identification of incompetent perforating veins is extremely difficult in the presence of healed ulceration or liposclerosis. There is also the risk of injecting sclerosant into the posterior tibial artery while attempting to sclerose incompetent perforating veins in the lower calf or ankle. Treatment of these veins by operation is therefore both more precise and reliable and is also safer than injection sclerotherapy.

Injection sclerotherapy

As in operative surgery, attention to detail is most important.

Technique
A modification of the collapsed vein technique introduced by Fegan in 1963[5] is used. The preferred sclerosant is sodium tetradecyl sulphate (STD) 3%.

1. The patient stands on a mounting block and the varices to be injected are carefully marked with a felt-tip pen (Figure 10.1).
2. The patient sits at the end of the examination couch with the legs hanging over the end. The surgeon sits opposite on a low chair. One or two pillows are placed halfway along the examination couch for the patient to lean back on. A good light is essential.
3. A No. 16 needle attached to a 2 ml syringe containing sclerosant is inserted into the vein. Care is taken that blood is drawn back into the syringe and that this is venous, e.g. dark in colour and non-pulsatile.
4. The patient leans backwards on the pillows, elevating the leg with help from an assistant. Two fingers of the surgeons left hand are placed above and below the needle to isolate a segment of vein about 5 cm long. Between 0.25 ml and 0.5 ml of sclerosant is then injected. A major error at this stage is to inject too great a quantity of solution; this does not ensure significantly better sclerosis and it does increase the risk of extravasation of sclerosant and subsequent skin ulceration.
5. A small cotton wool pad mounted on a 5 cm strip of Elastoplast is immediately applied by the assistant.
6. The patient then sits, lowering the legs, and the procedure is repeated on the next marked site. Large dilated varices can often be injected without the leg being lowered. A safe upper limit is 2 ml STD per leg per session. STD is nephrotoxic and care must be taken not to exceed the safe dose.
7. Immediately after the last injection, the leg is elevated and bandaged with a 10 or 15 cm elastocrepe bandage which is covered by Tubigrip stockinette. Some surgeons prefer medium compression (Class 2 compression) elastic stockings.
8. The patient is instructed to go immediately for a brisk walk; this is in order to clear excess sclerosant. The patient is advised to avoid prolonged standing and to walk briskly approximately three miles each day. There is no need to be obsessional about this, particularly as most women walk further than this

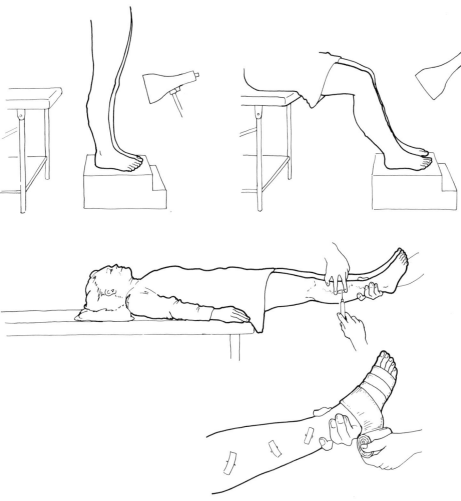

Figure 10.1 Injection sclerotherapy

distance in their day to day domestic duties. The patient is also advised to report to the clinic at once if the bandages become too loose, too tight or at all uncomfortable.

9. The patient attends the clinic again one week later. The bandages are removed, scurfy skin is washed away and the legs inspected. Residual varices are injected and cotton wool pads reapplied. Any lumpy thrombi are evacuated through small incisions under local anaesthesia, using a No. 11 blade. The legs are rebandaged, and the patient is seen once more in two weeks time. Fegan originally advised a total of six weeks bandaging, but a subsequent study[6] has shown that three weeks is sufficient.

Sensitivity reactions occasionally occur, usually at the second course of injections. Anaphylactic shock and death, though very rare, have been reported. Adrenaline, hydrocortisone, antihistamines and oxygen must always be available and the procedure must always be carried out in a properly organized clinic with a trained nurse or other experienced assistant.

There have been a number of reports of accidental injection into arteries[7], particularly into the posterior tibial artery, during attempts to sclerose incompetent perforating veins. *Always* draw blood back into the syringe and make certain that it is dark in colour and non-pulsatile; *never* inject if in any doubt whatsoever. Accidental intra-arterial injection has caused peripheral gangrene and loss of toes.

The surgical treatment of varicose veins

Surgery of the long saphenous vein
Shortly before the operation the patient must be examined after standing for several minutes in order to fill all varices. These are then marked with an indelible felt-tip pen. The long saphenous vein can usually be identified in the groin by means of the percussion test, thus enabling a short incision to be made over the saphenofemoral junction (see Figure 6.4, page 58).

The operation may be performed under general or epidural anaesthesia. Local anaesthesia is possible. This involves infiltration of the site of the groin incision by 1% lignocaine and also a femoral nerve block; the femoral artery is identified by its pulsation and the local anaesthetic is injected deeply lateral to this. The lateral cutaneous nerve of the thigh, which passes under the inguinal ligament just medial to the anterior superior iliac crest, must also be infiltrated with local anaesthetic. Epidural anaesthesia is usually a preferable option in patients who are unfit for general anaesthetic, and may be preferred by those who are fit. Bleeding is signficantly less with epidural than with inhalational anaesthesia.

The patient lies supine with the legs widely abducted on a padded board and with the operating table tilted head down (Figure 10.2). A skin crease incision is made 3 cm below the inguinal ligament, extending laterally for about 5 cm from the adductor longus origin. This landmark is easy to feel, even in the obese. The deep layer of superficial fascia (Scarpa's fascia) and a number of small blood vessels are divided and controlled by diathermy coagulation. The long saphenous vein is identified and followed to its termination at the foramen ovale where the superficial pudendal artery crosses beneath it (occasionally it crosses superficial to the long saphenous vein and the surgeon must be aware of this possibility). The tributaries are dissected, ligated and divided. Good retraction and good light are essential. More accidents occur at this stage of the operation than at any other; damage to the common femoral vein or even transection of the superficial femoral artery are all too comon. The usual reason is poor access and visibility and, in an obese patient or in any situation of difficulty, the wise surgeon will extend his incision.

The long saphenous vein is divided close to the saphenofemoral junction which is then ligated. Transfixion and ligation using a well-lubricated 2-0 black silk suture on a round-bodied needle is the safest procedure and avoids any risk of haemorrhage from a slipped ligature.

A Myers metal stripper or one of its modifications is passed down the long saphenous vein through its divided end and tied into place with a silk ligature. If competent valves are present in the upper part of the vein, the stripper will be unable to pass and the vein should then be simply ligated with a 2-0 chromic catgut suture. This technique of retrograde stripping avoids unnecessary stripping of a normal saphenous vein with competent valves and also indicates the length of vein which requires stripping. The stripper will normally pass down an incompetent long

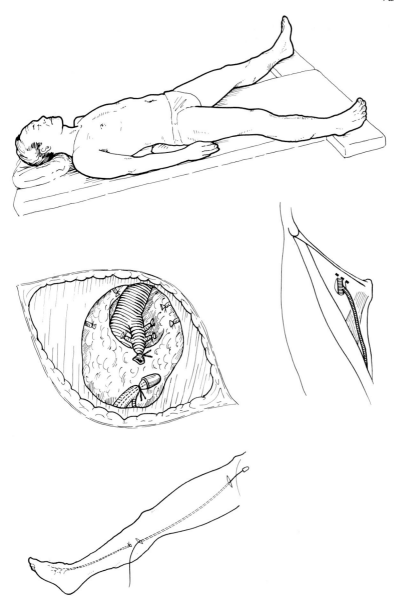

Figure 10.2 Surgery of the long saphenous vein

saphenous vein as far as the upper calf where its main varicose tributaries join it. Distal to this point most long saphenous veins are normal in diameter and their valves are competent; there is therefore no need to strip them. Avoiding interference with the normal distal long saphenous vein has two advantages: the normal segment of vein can be used for future coronary artery bypass grafting if required (cardiac surgeons do not like using varicose and dilated proximal saphenous veins) and damage to the saphenous nerve is avoided. The nerve lies about 1 cm away from the vein in the upper calf, but gradually becomes closer until it is intimately related at the ankle (see Figure 3.2, page 16). Stripping the distal saphenous vein is very likely to produce nerve damage, with resulting anaesthesia or parasthesiae on the anteromedial surface of the foot. The incidence of this complication varies from 23 to 58% in reported series[8-9]. By limiting the stripping operation to the proximal calf, the incidence is reduced to 4%[10].

There are those who question the need to strip the long saphenous vein at all, and advocate simple proximal division and ligation only. The argument in favour of stripping the thigh portion of the long saphenous vein is that this often communicates with the superficial femoral vein lying in the subsartorial (Hunter's) canal in the distal third of the thigh. Peroperative retrograde saphenography performed in a series of 60 patients demonstrated at least one hunterian perforating vein in 87% of 80 saphenograms[11]. Saphenofemoral ligation without stripping has a reported recurrence rate of 60%[8].

The most common complication of stripping the proximal long saphenous vein is severe haematoma formation in the thigh. Attempts to prevent this by tight bandaging are usually unsuccessful, as thigh bandages are notoriously prone to roll down and become ineffectual. This complication can largely be avoided by attaching a narrow suction drain (Redivac) with 30 cm of perforations to the stripper acorn immediately before the vein is stripped. A 3-0 silk stitch is used and this can be broken by a sharp pull when the Redicvac drain has been pulled down to knee level (Figure 10.3). The drain is removed after 24 or 48 hours, when drainage has ceased; between 50 and 100 ml blood is drained from most patients.

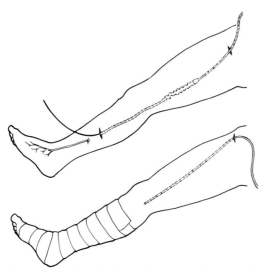

Figure 10.3 Redivac drainage of the long saphenous stripper track

Between performing the groin dissection and stripping the long saphenous vein, individual varices are avulsed through very small (2–3 mm) stab incisions made with a No. 11 blade (Figure 10.4). These incisions do not require suturing; they are closed with ¼ in (6 mm) Steristrips covered by Airstrip dressing. This technique

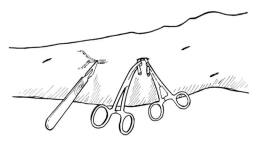

Figure 10.4 Avulsion of varices through small (2–3 mm) stab incisions. A No. 11 blade and mosquito forceps are used and the incisions are closed with Steristrips

avoids the tediousness of performing multiple fine sutures and the discomfort to the patient involved in their removal. The tiny incisions heal well and the long-term cosmetic result is excellent.

The groin incision is closed using interrupted 2-0 chromic catgut sutures to Scarpa's fascia and a subcuticular suture for the skin. The leg is then elevated and bandaged firmly with a crepe bandage from toes to thigh. The foot of the bed is elevated post-operatively but the patient is allowed to get up to wash and go to the lavatory, and short walks are encouraged after the first twelve hours. The crepe bandage is removed and replaced by a light (Class 1) compression stocking (Brevet or Kendal TED) 24 or 48 hours post-operatively. The patient is usually discharged, wearing elastic stockings, one or two days after simple long saphenous surgery; young and fit patients can undergo this surgery as day cases. Patients are usually fit to return to work two or three weeks after the operation.

Results
The results of the 'limited stripping' operation for long saphenous incompetence have been evaluated in 71 patients, with 96 operated legs, who were reviewed between two and a half and six years post-operatively[10]. Persistent or recurrent varicose veins were found in 14 legs of 12 patients (14.5%). Of these, 2 were the result of short saphenous incompetence which had developed since the operation for long saphenous stripping, 12 (12.5%) were therefore true long saphenous recurrences. Further surgery for recurrent varices of the long saphenous system was considered necessary in 4 legs, 8 legs of 6 patients being considered suitable for injection sclerotherapy. This compares with the reported recurrence rate of 60% following saphenofemoral ligation without stripping reported by Munn[8]. Paraesthesia or anaesthesia resulting from saphenous nerve damage was only found in 4% of patients.

Surgery of the short saphenous vein
Incompetence of the short saphenous vein may occur alone, but more often accompanies long saphenous incompetence. The two procedures are then carried out under the same anaesthetic. General anaesthesia is usual; intubation is required as the patient has to lie face downwards. Local anaestheisa is difficult, as this involves the need for sciatic nerve block; epidural anaesthesia is a suitable alternative.

Examination and preoperative vein marking are carried out as described for the long saphenous vein. The termination of the short saphenous vein is notoriously unreliable (see Chapter 3) and often difficult to feel by simple palpation. Hobbs[12] recommends 'on-table' short saphenous varicography in all patients. A simpler alternative is to use Doppler ultrasound examination, and with this the experienced surgeon can generally locate the saphenopopliteal junction accurately. Short saphenous varicography should be performed in any case of doubt, as failure to perform accurate saphenopopliteal ligation is very likely to result in recurrent varices.

The patient lies face downward with the chest and abdomen resting on a pillow (Figure 10.5). The popliteal fossa is explored through a 7–10 cm long skin crease

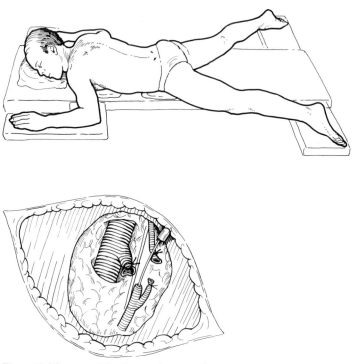

Figure 10.5 Surgery of the short saphenous vein

incision. Superficial vessels are controlled by diathermy and the deep fascia is opened in the line of the incision. The sural nerve is identified and preserved and the short saphenous vein is identified between the two heads of gastrocnemius. The *knee is flexed* by an assistant or by a sandbag placed under the leg (Figure 10.6). This important step enables thorough exploration of the popliteal fossa by relaxing the fascia lata and the gastrocnemius muscles. The vein is carefully traced through the popliteal fat towards its termination (feel for the pulsation of the popliteal artery). There is a constant tributary running along the posterior surface of the thigh (the residual post-axial vein) and other minor tributaries may need division and ligation; it is not usually necessary to divide the gastrocnemius veins. The short saphenous vein is ligated just superficial to the junction of the gastrocnemius veins, using 2-0 black silk. Opinion varies on whether the short saphenous vein should be

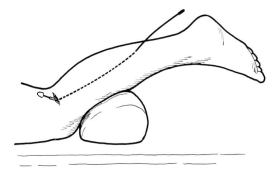

Figure 10.6 Short saphenous exploration in the popliteal fossa is considerably helped by flexing the knee

stripped or not. There is no constant equivalent to the hunterian perforating vein, which is the reason for stripping the long saphenous vein. However, there may be a midcalf perforating vein and, if the short saphenous vein is obviously dilated and incompetent, the author's practice is to strip it to the junction of the upper two-thirds and the lower third of the calf. As in the case of the long saphenous vein, more distal stripping may result in sural nerve damage and anaesthesia on the posterolateral surface of the heel and foot. Stripping is postponed until varices have been avulsed through stab incisions. Bandaging is performed as for long saphenous stripping, but suction drainage is unnecessary.

Venous ulceration

Venous ulceration is defined as ulceration of the malleolar skin in the presence of perforating vein incompetence, with or without deep vein incompetence. Perforating vein incompetence is often accompanied by saphenous incompetence. The 'venous' ulcer must be distinguished from the (uncommon) 'varicose' ulcer.

Venous ulcers are best treated by accurate diagnosis and surgical elimination of all points of venous reflux. Not all patients are suitable for surgery, which may be extensive, and alternatives are injection sclerotherapy or a combination of stanozolol or oxpentifylline and knee-length elastic compression stockings. Elastic stockings are also necessary to maintain long-term healing following surgery of saphenous and perforating veins in patients with deep vein incompetence and reflux. Elastic stockings alone, without either fibrinolytic enhancement or surgery, are usually ineffectual.

Surgery and elastic compression in the treatment of venous ulceration

The treatment of venous ulceration by perforating vein ligation was first popularised by Linton[13] and Cockett[14]. Following the latter's description of the anatomy of the direct perforating veins, and of the surgery required to ligate them, a number of carefully conducted studies of the results of perforating vein ligation were reported between 1961 and 1971. Altogether, over 1000 patients were followed for between five and nine years, with a success rate of about 90%[15–20]. However in the subsequent ten years, disappointing results were reported in patients with deep vein incompetence in addition to perforating vein incompetence[21–25]. In 1976 Burnand and his colleagues[22], undertook a retrospective study of 44 patients with venous ulceration who had been treated by direct perforating vein ligation five years previously. The state of the deep veins was investigated by ascending phlebography and, while they reported excellent results in those with normal deep veins, perforating vein ligation was invariably followed by recurrent ulceration in those with phlebographic evidence of damage to the deep veins. These observations were published shortly before the author became responsible for the venous ulcer clinic at Lewisham Hospital. Burnand's work suggested that there was some need to control residual venous hypertension after ligation of incompetent perforating veins in patients with deep venous incompetence. Valve transposition or replacement had not been described at that time and most of our patients were elderly and unfit for surgery of such complexity. It was therefore decided to attempt to control the calf venous hypertension resulting from popliteal reflux by elastic compression hosiery. Popliteal reflux and perforating vein incompetence was diagnosed by Doppler ultrasound examination, phlebography also being performed in 39 patients. Popliteal reflux was diagnosed in 44 legs of 32 patients and perforating vein incompetence in 108 of the 109 ulcerated legs. Saphenous incompetence was diagnosed in 36 patients and these veins were ligated and stripped at the same time as perforating vein ligation was performed. Most ulcers were healed before surgery, but where this was not achieved (in about 20%), skin grafting was performed at the same time as the venous surgery, with antibiotic cover. Post-operatively, all patients wore knee-length elastic compression (Class 2) stockings for two or three months until healing was complete. Those patients without deep venous incompetence were then advised that they need no longer wear compression hosiery, while those with popliteal reflux were advised to continue wearing knee-length stockings while ambulant, indefinitely.

The results of this policy have been encouraging. One of the original 77 patients died from metastatic squamous carcinoma in the immediate post-operative period, as a result of Marjolin's ulceration developing in the grafted ulcer. The results in the remaining 76 patients were initially assessed six years after the first patient was treated, 76% being followed up for more than three years. At that time 91 (84.3%) of the 108 ulcerated legs were healed and there was no difference between those patients with and without deep venous incompetence[1]. It became apparent that a large proportion of failures were patients with rheumatoid arthritis in addition to venous incompetence. There were 8 such patients with 12 ulcerated legs and they accounted for 9 of the 17 failures. When these 8 patients were excluded from the series, 88 of the 96 ulcerated legs (91.7%) remained healed. A second review has recently been completed, eleven years after the first patient was treated[26]. A number of patients were lost to follow-up, but a mean six-year follow-up rate was achieved. Seventy-three per cent of ulcers remain healed and there is no difference between those with perforating vein incompetence alone and those who also have deep venous incompetence. When patients with ischaemia and rheumatoid arthritis are excluded from this series, the ulcer healing rate improves to 80% in those with deep vein reflux and 84% in those with perforating vein incompetence alone.

It is uncertain why compression hosiery seems to improve the result of perforating and saphenous vein ligation in the treatment of venous ulceration. It has been suggested[27] that, following perforating vein ligation in patients with deep venous incompetence, the high intramuscular and deep venous pressure will continue to reach the superficial veins through residual perforating veins which are clinically undetectable. This hypothesis has never been substantiated by non-invasive investigations or by phlebography, and it is probably unnecessary to invoke the presence of mysterious and undetectable perforating veins. Careful examination of the corrosion cast dissection shown in Figure 3.6 (page 20), shows that the long saphenous vein communicates by two or three tributaries with the malleolar venous plexus (ankle venous flare veins) resulting from direct perforating vein incompetence. The distal long saphenous vein also communicates with the deep plantar veins through the communicating veins which join the dorsal venous arch between the metatarsals (Figure 3.3). Ligation of incompetent calf perforating veins and the proximal long saphenous vein are likely significantly to reduce venous hypertension in the ankle flare veins. However, in patients with deep venous incompetence the high deep venous pressures can still be transmitted to the malleolar veins through the distal long saphenous vein by way of the metatarsal perforating veins. Elastic compression hosiery may act mainly by compressing the long saphenous vein on the dorsum of the foot and anterior surface of the ankle and thus prevent the transmission of high venous pressures from deep to superficial ankle veins. It is logical to suppose that improved results in the treatment of venous ulceration might be achieved by an elasticated anklet or by ligation of the long saphenous vein distal to the malleolus; this hypothesis requires further investigation.

Surgery of the calf and ankle perforating veins
Accurate identification of the sites of perforating vein incompetence must be performed by examination and by Doppler ultrasound examination, and, if there remains any doubt, by ascending venography. A number of surgical approaches have been described, the most useful being those described by Linton, by Cockett and by Dodd.

Shearing and endoscopic procedures   A number of ingenious attempts have been made to interrupt incompetent perforating veins by avoiding a long incision through liposclerotic skin, with its poor healing properties. First described by Albanese[28], the instrument described by Edwards[29] is readily available and popular with some surgeons in the UK. The instrument and its use are illustrated in Figure 10.7. A small transverse incision is made on the medial surface of the calf well above the area of liposclerotic skin and is deepened to divide the deep fascia. The instrument is then passed down blindly between deep fascia and underlying muscles, traction being exerted on the handle in order to keep it as close to the deep fascia as possible. The aim is to shear through all perforating veins as they pass through the deep fascia to join the posterior tibial vein. The disadvantage of

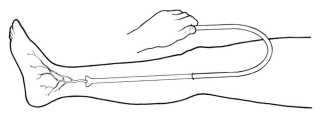

Figure 10.7 The Edwards phlebotome

this technique is that it is 'blind' and venograms must be performed before and after the procedure. This is necessary to make certain that all perforating veins are divided. Edwards has done this and has reported satisfactory results. Very firm bandaging must be applied during and after the use of the instrument if painful subfascial haematoma formation is to be avoided.

This instrument undoubtedly avoids the healing problems associated with long incisions through liposclerotic skin and shortens operating time. It is not without complications. In the author's experience, painful subfascial haematoma formation, probably resulting from inadequate bandaging, has led to a few dissatisfied patients. More seriously, use of the phlebotome in an elderly woman with very thin legs and friable skin resulted in an area of skin necrosis.

A number of ingenious attempts have been made to control incompetent perforating veins under direct vision but avoiding a long incision. The first involved the use of a Negus laryngoscope (designed over fifty years ago by the author's father, V. E. Negus, otolaryngologist, King's College Hospital, London), whose straight blade was passed subfascially through a high calf incision similar to that of a phlebotome. Traction on the blade, to elevate the deep fascia away from the muscles and illumination, was intended to demonstrate the incompetent perforating veins which could then be controlled by silver clips on a long applicator. The author's attempts to perform this apparently simple technique have been unsuccessful due to inadequate vision down the subfascial tunnel. A more promising approach has been made possible by the introduction of fibre-optic endoscopy, and a series of endoscopic tubes, through which coagulation forceps and scissors can be passed, have been described by Hower[30]. A similar instrument has recently been described by Fischer[31]. Acceptable results of endoscopic dissection of perforating veins have been reported by Jugenheimer and his colleagues[32].

The Linton operation   Linton[13] recommended thorough ligation of all perforating veins of the lower leg, anterior, lateral and medial, and described a subfascial approach to each. The anterior approach is no longer considered necessary and the long incisions which Linton described have also been rendered unnecessary by greater precision in identifying sites of perforating vein incompetence. The operation described here is therefore Cockett's[14] modification of Linton's subfascial approach to the medial incompetent direct perforating veins. The sites of perforating vein incompetence are established by the methods which have been described and marked on the skin with indelible ink. The incision lies over these, usually 2.5–5 cm posterior to the posterior border of the tibia (Figure 10.8). If one perforating vein only requires ligation, a 5 cm incision should be sufficient. In the very fat leg this may need to be longer. If there are two or more perforating veins, the incision is made over all of them, extending 2.5 cm further in each direction. Superficial fat and deep fascia are divided and the incompetent perforating veins are identified as they pass through gaps in the deep fascia, close to the posterior border of the tibia, to join the posterior tibial vein. An incompetent perforating vein is usually 3 mm or more in diameter. Turner-Warwick's bleed back test can be performed to demonstrate incompetence after making a small incision in the vein wall. The vein or veins are then ligated and divided, the deep fascia is closed with interrupted 2-0 catgut sutures and the skin is loosely closed with interrupted nylon or Prolene sutures. The wound is dressed with a soft dressing; we have found Mepore very acceptable. Elasticated waterproof dressings may become too tight,

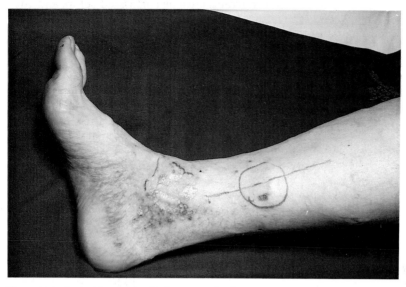

Figure 10.8 The incision for the Cockett operation for perforating vein ligation

particularly if encrusted with blood, and lead to pain in the post-operative period. Firm bandaging, followed by medium compression (Class 2) stockings, is necessary for two or three weeks post-operatively, during which time the leg must be elevated. These incisions are notoriously slow to heal and sutures must be left in place much longer than is necessary for the groin or popliteal incisions. The wound is inspected one week to ten days post-operatively and half the sutures are usually removed at this stage, the remainder being removed one week later.' With these precautions, wound dehiscence rarely occurs.

The modified Linton subfascial approach can also be used to divide incompetent lateral perforating veins, the incision then being placed just posterior to the fibula.

The Cockett operation   Cockett[14] described the extrafascial division and ligation of incompetent calf perforating veins. The straight incision lies one finger's breadth behind and parallel to the posterior border of the tibia (Figure 10.8). Starting nearly halfway up the leg, it is extended to a point one inch above and behind the medial malleolus. The incision is carried straight down to the deep fascia, where lateral dissection can be safely carried out in that plane. The perforators are identified and ligated at their points of entry into the foramina in the deep fascia.

The Dodd operation   While the Linton and Cockett operations provide excellent access to the direct calf perforating veins, lipodermatosclerosis of the overlying skin and subcutaneous fat is a common complication of incompetence of these veins, and incisions made through this skin heal very poorly indeed, with a significant incidence of wound dehiscence and infection. The problem is exacerbated by the relatively poor arteriolar supply of this area, derived from small perforating arteries[33]. The posteromedial subfascial approach, described by Dodd in 1964[34], avoids both medial and lateral indurated areas. Good access is afforded to the

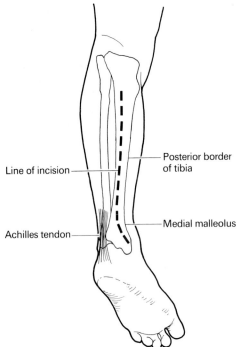

Line of incision

Posterior border
of tibia

Medial malleolus

Achilles tendon

Figure 10.9 Dodd's posteromedial incision for
perforating vein ligation

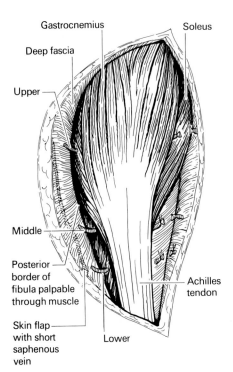

Gastrocnemius

Soleus

Deep fascia

Upper

Middle

Posterior
border of
fibula palpable
through muscle

Achilles
tendon

Skin flap
with short
saphenous
vein

Lower

Figure 10.10 After division of the deep fascia in the
line of incision (Figure 10.9), the muscles can be
retracted, first laterally and then medially, to
expose medial and lateral perforating veins

medial and lateral perforating veins and the incision heals well. This incision is preferable to the posterior mid-line 'stocking seam' incision as the latter may result in painful tethering of skin to the Achilles tendon.

The patient is intubated and placed face downwards, as for short saphenous surgery. The incision is placed 2.5 cm medial to the midline and the lower end is swung still more medially in order to avoid the Achilles tendon (Figure 10.9). Avoiding the sural nerve, the deep fascia is incised along the length of the incision. By retracting the bellies of gastrocnemius laterally and then medially, the subfascial compartment is opened sufficiently to identify the medial and lateral direct perforating veins (Figure 10.10). These are either divided and ligated, or ligated in continuity using 2-0 black silk on an aneurysm needle. The late Harold Dodd used to emphasise the importance of always 'getting down to bone'; that is, always dissect between the muscles and the deep fascia until reaching the medial border of the tibia. By doing this, it is impossible to miss any perforating veins communicating with the posterior tibial vein. They are often hidden in the medial intermuscular septum and can be difficult to find. The deep fascia is closed with interrupted 2-0 chromic catgut sutures and the skin is closed with interrupted nylon sutures. The leg is firmly bandaged with a crepe bandage. Subfascial exploration of perforating veins has a high risk of post-operative deep vein thrombosis and prophylaxis by subcutaneous heparin, 5000 units 12-hourly, until the patient's discharge is most important.

Aftercare is as for the Linton and Cockett operations, with slow mobilisation, prolonged firm compression bandaging or stockings and delayed removal of sutures.

Results
The results of calf perforating vein ligation in the treatment of venous ulceration have been described in the introductory paragraphs to this section (page 133). The long-term results of this surgery are difficult to evaluate as most of the patients are elderly and a significant proportion have atherosclerotic arterial insufficiency. In some cases, there was no evidence of ischaemia at the time of the perforating vein ligation or at the first review between one and six years post-operatively; however, at the second review, five years later, it was evident that deterioration in the arterial blood supply had progressed to the extent that ischaemia was contributing significantly to ulcer recurrence. In spite of this, over 70% of ulcers remained healed following the policy of perforating vein ligation, with saphenous ligation and stripping where necessary; patients with Doppler ultrasound evidence of popliteal reflux being advised to wear knee-length Class 2 compression stockings during their waking hours. Exclusion of patients with rheumatoid arthritis or ischaemia improved the ulcer-free rate to over 80%. It has been remarked that one of the more remarkable features of this study was patient compliance, in that they continued to adhere to advice to wear compression stockings. This is in marked contrast to the findings of Chant and his colleagues[35]. It seems likely that patient co-operation was largely related to the fact that most of these patients had suffered many years of recurrent ulceration as a result of conservative treatment. They were therefore keen to co-operate in their own treatment as far as they were able.

This point is mentioned as the need for co-operation and involvement in his or her own treatment must be emphasized to each patient at the first attendance at the ulcer clinic and repeated from time to time at subsequent attendances. We have not found this an arduous task. Most South London patients are only too happy to do whatever they can to help themselves and this has undoubtedly been an important factor in achieving good results. Patients in other areas may be less co-operative.

Surgery of other perforating veins

Apart from the calf perforating veins, which by transmitting high venous pressures from the deep compartment of the leg to the malleolar flare veins would appear to be most important in the aetiology of venous ulceration, there are other, less common, perforating veins which may contribute to varicose veins and superficial venous insufficiency. These are the medial tibial tubercle perforator (Boyd's perforator), which communicates directly with the long saphenous vein, the less common lateral tibial tubercle perforator, the gastrocnemius perforator, which may communicate with the short saphenous vein, the hunterian perforators which join the superficial femoral vein in the distal subsartorial canal to the long saphenous vein in 87% of patients[11], and the very rare upper lateral thigh or tensor fascia lata perforators. These can be detected by venography or Doppler ultrasound examination and treated either by injection sclerotherapy or by ligation through small incisions similar to the Cockett incision for the calf perforators. It is sometimes necessary to divide the hunterian thigh perforating veins through such an incision, usually in the treatment of recurrent varicose veins following inadequate long saphenous surgery. This operation should not be necessary if the long saphenous vein is stripped to distal thigh or upper calf level as described. As these perforating veins, unlike the calf perforating veins, communicate directly with the long saphenous vein, saphenous stripping to below this level will effectively avulse them, making direct surgery unnecessary.

Surgery of deep venous reflux

Deep venous reflux, usually post-thrombotic, is a most important factor in the aetiology of venous ulceration. Following calf perforating vein ligation, recurrent ulceration is inevitable in the presence of venographic evidence of deep vein damage[22]. In the author's clinic, where most patients are elderly and we are anxious to limit venous surgery to the minimum, deep venous reflux is usually controlled by the use of knee-length Class 2 compression stockings. In recent years a number of ingenious operations have been developed, mainly in the USA.

Operations to prevent deep venous reflux may be divided into four groups: (1) deep vein ligation, (2) 'sling' operations, (3) valve repairs, and (4) valve transposition or transplantation.

Deep vein ligation   The first attempts to control deep venous reflux were by ligating either the superficial femoral or popliteal vein in the mistaken belief that reflux alone was responsible for post-thrombotic symptoms and signs[36]. Post-thrombotic deep venous obstruction is now well-recognised to be associated with severe 'bursting' pain on walking (venous claudication) and it is not surprising that surgical ligation of the deep veins was unsuccessful.

Sling operations   An ingenious attempt to prevent reflux down the popliteal vein during calf muscle relaxation has been described by Psathakis[37]. He detached the tendon of gracillis so that it formed a sling round the vein. The operation has subsequently been modified by the use of a Silastic sling. Psathakis has reported encouraging results, but as yet these have not been confirmed by other surgeons and the operation is not often performed.

Valve repair operations   Several ingenious procedures have been described to repair or plicate floppy and incompetent valves in the deep veins[38]. These are unfortunately not applicable to patients with post-thrombotic deep venous incompetence, in which thrombus recanalisation and retraction has usually damaged the valves beyond hope of repair. Congenital absence of valves or floppy incompetent valves are extremely rare conditions[39]; few cases are likely to be encountered in a typical ulcer clinic.

Valve transposition and valve transplantation operations   Attempts have been made to restore some valve function to incompetent superficial femoral veins by anastomosing the upper part of this vein to a segment of proximal long saphenous vein containing at least one competent valve. Ferris and Kistner[40] reported encouraging results, phlebograms performed three years post-operatively indicating that reflux had been restored to normal in most patients. However Queral and his colleagues' long-term results[41] were less encouraging; immediately post-operatively, post-exercise foot vein pressure recovery time had returned to normal limits but, twelve months later, the mean recovery time had become abnormal again and nine patients had developed recurrent ulcers.

An alternative approach has been devised by Taheri *et al.*[42], whose operation involves resecting a segment of axillary vein containing a competent valve and suturing this into the post-thrombotic and incompetent popliteal vein. The operation is not technically difficult; the axillary vein can be exposed without difficulty by splitting the upper fibres of pectoralis major, and collateral veins from the arm, particularly the cephalic vein, protect against the development of hand or arm oedema. Results have been a little more encouraging than the valve transposition operations and Taheri has reported clinical improvement in 32 of 43 limbs. Objective measurements of venous function have been disappointingly few, and Raju[43], in describing the results of 22 valve transplants, has concluded that these tend to deteriorate with the passage of time. It is perhaps not surprising that a single valve, transplanted into an incompetent deep venous system, is not likely to withstand the high venous pressures for very long.

The author's experience is confined to only one patient with bilateral deep venous incompetence and severe ankle ulceration which had persisted in spite of extensive surgery to ligate incompetent perforating and saphenous veins. The Taheri operation was performed without difficulty in one leg, but failed to achieve any detectable improvement of the ulcer. Similar surgery to the second leg was not considered justified and the patient continues to be treated by dressings and compression bandaging.

Summary

It is disappointing that so many ingenious efforts to restore valvular function to the deep veins have shown poor or at best indifferent long-term results. Those starting out on the treatment of venous ulceration should limit their surgery to perforating vein ligation and saphenous ligation and stripping, with advice to patients with popliteal reflux to wear knee-length firm compression stockings when ambulant post-operatively. If this management is felt insufficient, either stanozolol or oxpentifylline may be added. Operations for correcting deep venous reflux may still be indicated in those in whom more simple measures have proved ineffectual. At the present time, there is little to choose in the published results between the Psathakis Silastic sling procedure and Taheri's axillary vein valve transposition. Development of this surgery is in its very early stages and those with an interest in the management of venous ulceration would be well advised to keep a careful eye on the literature where, hopefully, more encouraging long-term results may be published in the next few years.

Surgery of venous obstruction

Deep vein stenosis or occlusion, resulting in obstruction to venous return from the leg, is considerably less common than deep venous incompetence. By contrast, operations for its relief, at least as far as iliac vein obstruction is concerned, are rather more successful.

Deep venous obstruction most commonly affects the iliac veins, usually the left, and most often follows massive iliofemoral venous thrombosis. It may also result from compression from malignant lymph nodes, perivenous fibrosis following radiotherapy or from the pressure of an iliac aneurysm. Post-thrombotic occlusion of the superficial femoral vein is far less common than that of the iliac veins and is usually adequately compensated by an increase in the deep venous blood flow along the profunda femoris vein and long saphenous vein. Operations for this condition are therefore rarely indicated and are generally less successful than surgery for the relief of iliac vein obstruction.

Iliac vein obstruction
The left common iliac vein is most commonly affected, for reasons which have been described in Chapter 3. Pre-existing narrowing and intraluminal band formation at the termination of the left common iliac vein predisposes to iliofemoral thrombosis and also inhibits post-thrombotic recanalisation. The patient usually presents with a swollen lower limb, and dilated groin collateral veins may be visible. Venous claudication, 'bursting pain' in the calf after walking a short distance, is of particular diagnostic significance. Investigation by perfemoral venography will demonstrate the site of occlusion and also dilated collateral veins, particularly through the uterine circulation. Venography is unable to indicate whether these collaterals are sufficiently numerous and dilated to compensate for the main iliac venous obstruction, and further investigation, by plethysmographic venous outflow measurement, or preferably (in the author's view) femoral venous pressure measurement, is necessary. Normal femoral venous pressures in the horizontal position are between 8 and 10 mmHg and do not rise more than 2 mmHg on exercise of the limb. Proximal venous obstruction greatly increases this rise in exercising venous pressure and an exercising femoral venous pressure of 22 mmHg was recently recorded in a 17-year-old boy suffering from post-thrombotic occlusion of the left common iliac vein.

Early attempts at direct surgery of the occluded vein included dissection of the vein from its constrictive perivenous fibrous tissue[44], veno-venoplasty to dilate the occluded segment, and attempts to prevent continued pressure of the right common iliac artery on the common iliac vein by means of plastic bridges. All these operations involve major abdominal surgery and a hazardous dissection. They have largely been abandoned and have been superseded by the operation of femorofemoral vein bypass using the contralateral long saphenous vein, which was first described by Palma and Esperon in 1959[45].

Under general anaesthesia, the patient lies supine on the operating table with the legs widely abducted. The right long saphenous vein is mobilised to just above the knee, all branches being meticulously ligated with fine black silk as for a femoropopliteal arterial reconstruction. The left common femoral vein and artery are exposed through a groin incision. This can be a very difficult dissection due to the presence of numerous wide, thin-walled collateral veins communicating with the saphenofemoral junction. A subcutaneous tunnel is fashioned through the suprapubic fat and the right long saphenous vein is pulled through this and anastomosed side-to-side to the left common femoral vein using continuous 6-0 Prolene sutures (Figure 10.11). Complete mobilisation of the femoral vein is not

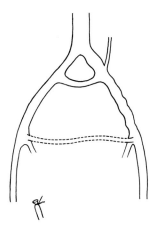

Figure 10.11 The Palma operation for iliac vein occlusion

usually necessary as sufficient control can generally be obtained by the use of a Satinsky partial occlusion clamp. The end of the long saphenous vein, or a tributary, if one is conveniently available, is then anastomosed end-to-side to the common femoral artery. A loop of nylon is placed round this arteriovenous anastomosis, its ends being passed through a metal button buried in the subcutaneous fat. The wounds are closed in layers, with suction drainage. The arteriovenous fistula is closed between two and three months post-operatively by locating the button by pre-operative X-ray. This is then dissected out of the often dense scar tissue and the nylon suture is gently tightened to occlude the fistula. Patency of the graft and pulsation from the arteriovenous fistula can usually be detected by means of a hand-held Doppler probe. Doppler ultrasound is also useful in ensuring that the arteriovenous fistula is successfully closed at the second operation. Full anticoagulation is not usually necessary when an arteriovenous fistula has been fashioned, but the patient receives 'microdose' intravenous heparin (1000 units 12-hourly) during the immediate post-operative period. This small dose of heparin has been demonstrated to have an antiplatelet effect[46], which helps to maintain patency of the arteriovenous fistula, and is also effective in the prevention of deep venous thrombosis[47].

If no suitable saphenous vein is available, ring-reinforced PTFE may be used as an alternative. It is essential to add an arteriovenous fistula and results are not as good as with the use of autogenous vein. However, recent reports have shown graft patency rates of between 20 and 100%, with a mean of 66%, and where the saphenous vein is absent or inadequate, ringed PTFE with a temporary arteriovenous fistula and prolonged anticoagulation provides an alternative.

The results of the Palma operation have been collected by Eklöf and Juhan[48]; they found a mean 78% success rate in five series (446 operations) in which autogenous saphenous vein was used. In a further five series (44 operations) using synthetic materials, the mean success rate was 67%. The author's results are similar, with a 73% patency rate in 11 operations. Two of these operations were performed in the same patient; following occlusion of a saphenous vein graft, a PTFE graft was inserted, with an arteriovenous fistula. The second graft remains patent three months post-operatively. Two other patients, in whom the saphenous graft was demonstrated to have occluded, declined further surgery, saying that their symptoms were not severe. This illustrates the difficulty of long-term follow-up in these cases. It would seem that venous collateral development can continue for several years after the acute thrombosis and it is likely that this is the reason for improvement in these two patients, in spite of occlusion of their grafts.

Femoral vein occlusion
Post-thrombotic occlusion of the superficial femoral vein is considerably less common than iliac venous obstruction. Even when ascending venography demonstrates occlusion of the superficial femoral vein, dilatation of collateral veins, particularly the profunda femoris, usually prevents any significant obstruction to venous return from the lower leg. It is important therefore to supplement venography with functional evaluation of venous blood flow, either by foot venous pressure measurement or calf plethysmography.

The operation of popliteal-femoral bypass was first described by Warren and Thayer in 1954[49] and subsequently by Husni[50], May[51] and Frileaux *et al.*[52].

With the patient lying supine under general anaesthesia and the legs widely abducted, the saphenous vein is exposed immediately posterior to the medial border of the tibia and its tributaries are divided and ligated using fine silk. The deep fascia is incised and the popliteal vein exposed and mobilised. The long saphenous vein is divided in the upper third of the calf and the distal end is ligated with chromic catgut. The proximal end is anastomosed end-to-side to the popliteal vein, using 6-0 Prolene (Figure 10.12). Gruss[53] modified the operation in 1975 by

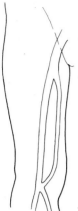

Figure 10.12 The Warren–Husni operation for occlusion of the superficial femoral vein

Diagnosis and treatment of venous ulceration

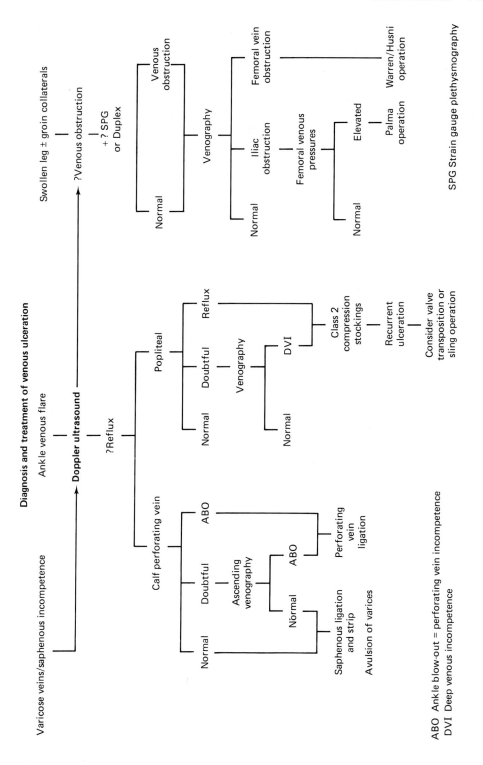

ABO Ankle blow-out = perforating vein incompetence
DVI Deep venous incompetence

SPG Strain gauge plethysmography

adding a peripheral arteriovenous anastomosis, using a side-to-side saphenopo-pliteal anastomosis and using the distal few centimetres of the saphenous vein to perform an end-to-side anastomosis to the posterior tibial artery. Gruss recommends magnification and 8-0 monofilament sutures for the arteriovenous anastomosis. Tight compression bandaging is avoided if an arteriovenous anastomosis has been used, as this may occlude the anastomosis. It is finally occluded two or three months after the first operation by applying a tight compression bandage; Gruss has only had to operate to close the anastomosis in three of his eight cases.

Results
There are few results reported in the literature and these indicate that the patency rate is significantly less than that of the Palma operation. Gruss has described the results in twelve patients, in whom arteriovenous fistula was performed in eight. In this series, three of the twelve saphenopopliteal bypasses thrombosed, with recurrence of symptoms. In a further four patients, calf muscle pump function demonstrated by foot venous pressure measurement was found to have deteriorated in spite of patent bypasses. Gruss does not indicate whether his successful bypasses were those with arteriovenous fistulae or not. May has reported the late results of seven patients, of whom four had improved and three had deteriorated. Husni[54] has reported a 66% patency rate in twenty-five cases, and the results of Frileaux et al.[52] in twenty patients are similar.

This author's extremely small experience of two patients has been disappointing. In one patient the popliteal vein was found to be densely occluded with organised thrombus, through which there were numerous very small recanalisation channels, an appearance similar to that of the muzzle of a Gatling gun. The operation was abandoned. In the second case, end-to-side saphenopopliteal anastomosis was performed to a patent popliteal vein without any difficulty; arteriovenous anastomosis was not performed. The patient was maintained on full warfarin anticoagulation and the graft remained patent for six months. At the end of this time, it suddenly and spontaneously thrombosed, in spite of adequate anticoagulation. Shortly afterwards an inoperable cerebral tumour was diagnosed and the patient died a few months later.

References

1. Negus, D., Friedgood, A. The effective management of venous ulceration. *Br. J. Surg.* **70**: 623–625, 1983
2. Callam, M. J., Harper, D. R., Dale, J. J., Ruckley, C. V. Chronic ulcer of the leg: clinical history. *Br. Med J.* **294**: 1389–1391, 1987
3. Cornwall, J. V., Dore, C. J., Chadwick, S. T. D., Lewis, J. D. Leg ulcers resurrected – a seven year follow-up. Paper read to Venous Forum Meeting, Manchester, May 1989
4. Hobbs, J. T. The treatment of varicose veins; a random trial of injection–compression therapy versus surgery. *Br. J. Surg.* **55**: 777–780, 1968
5. Fegan, W. G. Continuous compression technique of injecting varicose veins. *Lancet* **2**: 109–112, 1963
6. Reddy, P., Terry, T., Lamont, P., Dormandy, J. What is the correct duration of bandaging following sclerotherapy? In *Phlebology '85* (eds Negus, D., Jantet, G.), London, Libbey, pp. 141–142, 1986
7. MacGowan, W. A. L. Sclerotherapy: prevention of accidents. A review. *J. R. Soc. Med.* **78**: 136–137, 1985

8. Munn, S. R., Morton, J. B., Macbeth, W. A. A. G., McLeish, A. R. To strip or not to strip the long saphenous vein? A varicose veins trial. *Br. J. Surg.* **68**: 426–428, 1981

9. Cox, S. J., Wellwood, J. M., Martin, A. Saphenous nerve injury caused by stripping of the long saphenous vein. *Br. Med. J.* **1**: 415–417, 1974

10. Negus, D., Nichols, R. W. T. Is it necessary to strip the incompetent saphenous vein to the ankle? In *Phlebology '85* (eds Negus D., Jantet, G.), London, Libbey, pp. 148–150, 1986

11. Sutton, R., Darke, S. G. Should the long saphenous vein be stripped? A study by peroperative retrograde saphenography. In *Phlebology '85* (eds Negus, D., Jantet, G.), London, Libbey pp. 196–199, 1986

12. Hobbs, J. T. Per-operative venography to ensure accurate saphenopopliteal vein ligation. *Br. Med. J.* **2**: 1578–1579, 1980

13. Linton, R. R. Post-thrombotic ulceration of the lower extremity: its aetiology and surgical management. *Ann. Surg.* **107**: 582–593, 1938

14. Cockett, F. B. Pathology and treatment of venous ulcers. *Thesis,* University of London, 1953

15. Cranley, J. J., Krause, R. S., Strasser, E. S. Chronic venous insufficiency of the lower extremity. *Surgery* **49**: 48–58, 1961

16. Hansson, L. O. Venous ulcers of the lower limb. *Acta Chir. Scand.* **128**: 269–277, 1964

17. Bertelsen, S., Gammelgaard, A. Surgical treatment of post-thrombotic leg ulcers. *J. Cardiovasc. Surg.* **6**: 452–455, 1965

18. Silver, D., Gleysteen, J. J., Rhodes, G. R., *et al.* Surgical treatment of the refractory post-thrombotic ulcers. *Arch. Surg.* **103**: 544–560, 1971

19. Field, P., van Boxall, P. The role of the Linton flap procedure in the management of stasis dermatitis and ulceration in the lower limb. *Surgery* **70**: 920–926, 1971

20. Arnoldi, C. C., Haeger, K. Ulcus cruris venosum – crux medicorum? *Läkartidningen* **64**: 2149–2157, 1967

21. Recek, E. A critical appraisal of the role of ankle perforators for the genesis of venous ulcers in the lower leg. *J. Cardiovasc. Surg.* **12**: 45–49, 1971

22. Burnand, K. G., Lea Thomas, M., O'Donnell, E., Browse, N. L. The relation between post-phlebitic changes in the deep veins and the results of surgical treatment of venous ulcers. *Lancet* **1**: 936–938, 1976

23. Strandness, D. E., Thiele, D. L. *Selected Topics in Venous Disorders,* New York, Futura, 1981

24. Lumley, J. S. P. Surgical treatment of varicose veins. In *Contemporary Operative Surgery* (ed. Marsden, A.), London, Northwood Books, p. 184, 1979

25. Browse, N. L., Burnand, K. G. The causes of venous ulceration. *Lancet* **2**: 243–245, 1982

26. Holme, T. C., Negus, D. The treatment of venous ulceration by surgery and elastic compression hosiery; a long-term review. In *Phlebology* **5**: 125–128, 1990

27. Bjordal, R. I. Pressure and flow measurements in venous insufficiency of the legs. In *Controversies in the Management of Venous Disorders* (eds Eklöf, B., Gjöres, J. E., Thulesius, O., Bergqvist, D.), London, Butterworths, p. 34, 1989

28. Albanese, A. R. Escoplage: a new surgical technique for the treatment of varicose veins in the legs. *J. Cardiovasc. Surg.* **6**: 491–494, 1965

29. Edwards, J. M. Shearing operation for incompetent perforating veins. *Br. J. Surg.* **63**: 885–886, 1976

30. Hower, G. Operative technique of the endoscopic subfascial dissection of perforating veins. *Chirurg* **58**: 172–175, 1987

31. Fischer, R. Surgical treatment of varicose veins; endoscopic treatment of incompetent Cockett veins. In *Phlébologie '89* (eds Davy, A., Stemmer, R.), Paris, Libbey, p. 1040, 1989

32. Jugenheimer, M., Nagel, K., Junginger, T. Endoscopical sectioning of perforating veins. In *Phlébologie' 89* (eds Davy, A., Stemmer, R.), Paris, Libbey, pp. 1038–1039, 1989

33. Dodd, H., Cockett, F. B. *The Pathology and Surgery of the Veins of the Lower Limb,* 2nd edn, Edinburgh, Churchill Livingstone, p. 49, 1976

34. Dodd, H. The diagnosis and ligation of incompetent perforating veins. *Ann. R. Coll. Surg. Engl.* **34**: 186–196, 1964

35. Chant, A. D. B., Davies, L. J., Pike, J. M., Sparks, M. J. Support stockings in practical management of varicose veins. *Phlebology* **4**: 167–169, 1989

36. Bauer, G. Division of the popliteal vein in the treatment of so-called varicose ulceration. *Br. Med. J.* **2**: 318, 1950

37. Psathakis, N. Has the 'substitute valve' at the popliteal vein solved the problem of venous insufficiency of the lower extremity? *J. Cardiovasc. Surg.* **9**: 64–70, 1968

38. Kistner, R. L. Surgical repair of the incompetent femoral vein valves. *Arch. Surg.* **110**: 1336–1342, 1975

39. Eriksson, I. Vein valve surgery for deep valvular incompetence. In *Controversies in the Management of Venous Disorders* (eds Eklöf, B., Gjöres, J. E., Thulesius, O., Bergqvist, D.), London, Butterworths, pp. 267–268, 1989

40. Ferris, E. B., Kistner, R. L. Femoral vein reconstruction in the management of chronic venous insufficiency. *Arch. Surg.* **117**: 1571–1579, 1982

41. Queral, L. A., Whitehouse, W. M., Flinn, W. R., Neiman, H. L., Yao, J. S. T., Bergan, J. J. Surgical correction of chronic deep venous insufficiency by valvular transposition. *Surgery* **87**: 688–695, 1980

42. Taheri, S. A., Heffner, R., Meenaghan, M. A., *et al.* Technique and results of venous valve transplantation. In *Surgery of the Veins* (eds Bergan, J. J., Yao, J. S. T.), Orlando, Grune and Stratton, p. 219, 1985

43. Raju, S. Venous insufficiency of the lower limb and stasis ulceration. *Ann. Surg.* **197**: 688–697, 1983

44. Wanke, R., Gumrich, H. Chronische Beckenvenensperre. *Zentralbl. Chir.* **75**: 1302–1312, 1950

45. Palma, E. C., Esperon, R. Tratamiento del sindrome post thromboflebitico mediante transplante de safena interna. *Angiologia* **11**: 87–94, 1959

46. Negus, D., Pinto, D. J., Slack, W. W. The effect of small doses of heparin on platelet adhesiveness and lipoprotein-lipase activity before and after surgery. *Lancet* **1**: 1202–1204, 1971

47. Negus, D., Friedgood, A. Micro-dose intravenous heparin in the prevention of post-operative deep vein thrombosis. In *Phlebology '85* (eds Negus, D., Jantet, G.), London, Libbey, pp. 402–403, 1986

48. Eklöf, B., Juhan, C. Venous compression syndrome caused by anatomical anomalies. In *Controversies in the Management of Venous Disorders* (eds Eklöf, B., Gjöres, J. E., Thulesius, O. Bergquvist, D.), London, Butterworths, p. 297, 1989

49. Warren, R., Thayer, T. Transplantation of the saphenous vein for post-phlebitic stasis. *Surgery* **35**: 867–876, 1954

50. Husni, E. A. *In situ* saphenopopliteal bypass graft for incompetence of the femoral and popliteal veins. *Surg. Gynecol. Obstet.* **130**: 279–284, 1970

51. May, R. *Surgery of the Veins of the Leg and Pelvis*, Philadelphia, Saunders, p. 150, 1979

52. Frileaux, C., Pillot-Bienayme, P., Gillot, C. Bypass of segmental obliterations of ilio-femoral venous axis by transposition of the saphenous vein. *J. Cardiovasc. Surg.* **13**: 409–414, 1972

53. Gruss, J. D. Zur Modifikation des Femoralisbypass nach May. *Vasa* **4**: 59–61, 1975

54. Husni, E. A. Clinical experience through femoropopliteal venous reconstruction. In *Venous Problems* (eds Bergen, J. J., Yao, S. T.), Chicago, Year Book Medical Publishers, p. 485, 1978

Chapter 11

The treatment of ischaemic and other leg ulcers; recurrent ulceration

Ischaemic ulceration

Ischaemic ulcers may result from small vessel disease, atherosclerotic occlusion of the main limb arteries, or from a combination of both. Vasculitic ulcers will be considered separately below.

Many patients with ischaemic ulceration arrive in the clinic with a letter requesting treatment of an intractable 'venous ulcer' and with tight bandages conscientiously applied by a district nurse. It is obviously important that these are removed and replaced by light crepe bandages. An appropriately tactful letter then has to be composed to the general practitioner and his hardworking nurses to avoid repetition of tight compression.

Complete investigation of an ischaemic ulcer depends on arteriography, and theoretically this should be performed in every case, on the principle that treatment should always be based on accurate diagnosis. However, as many of these patients are very old and unfit for direct arterial surgery, it is often more sensible to try to obtain ulcer healing by conservative measures before proceeding to invasive investigations.

Patients with a palpable popliteal pulse, even those sufficiently young and fit for surgical treatment, are unlikely to be suitable for direct arterial surgery but may respond favourably to chemical lumbar sympathectomy or prostacyclin treatment followed by skin grafting.

It is often thought that the presence of one ankle pulse indicates adequate blood supply to the foot and ankle so that any ulceration is likely to be ischaemic in origin. This is a dangerous assumption and the author has experience of three patients who presented with supramalleolar ulceration, apparently of venous origin. In each case only one ankle or foot pulse could be felt or detected by Doppler ultrasound, and examination and further investigation showed no evidence of venous disorder. These patients' ulcers all healed following chemical lumbar sympathectomy.

Conservative treatment

Bed rest, dressings and antibiotics
Bed rest and good nursing in hospital, with daily dressings and appropriate antibiotics for infected ulcers, will often effect remarkable improvement, particularly in the elderly and in those on low income and in poor housing. Dressings should consist of one layer of non-adhesive dry dressing covered by

absorbent cotton gauze and kept in place by a *lightly applied* crepe bandage. Elevating the head of the bed may assist blood flow to the foot, but in the elderly this can result in unacceptable oedema and require a return to the horizontal position. Appropriate antibiotics should be prescribed after obtaining a swab result. Warm conditions and good food undoubtedly assist healing. Oxpentifylline (Trental) 400 mg t.d.s. may be helpful and cigarette smoking *must* be stopped.

Lumbar sympathectomy

Lumbar sympathectomy has been demonstrated to produce a 10% increase in capillary skin blood flow[1] and, in one series, was demonstrated to relieve ischaemic rest pain in 83% of 36 patients and to heal 50% of 52 trophic lesions[2]. Chemical lumbar sympathectomy, by the injection of phenol in water around the lumbar sympathetic chain, with the help of image intensifier radiography, is less traumatic than the operative procedure and it has been suggested that its effects are more durable than those obtained by surgical denervation[2]. Chemical sympathectomy has the additional advantage of avoiding the need for admission to hospital. Sympathectomy is usually ineffectual in patients with ankle pulse pressures less than 30 mmHg or an ankle:brachial index less than 0.25[3]. It is also usually ineffectual in diabetics. It is most important to establish that the ulcer is truly ischaemic before recommending sympathectomy; Linton described 'serious post-sympathectomy complications' in some patients with the post-thrombotic syndrome who were treated by lumbar sympathectomy[4].

Prostacyclin

The effectiveness of prostacyclin (epoprostenol, Flolan; Wellcome) in the treatment of ischaemic ulcers was first demonstrated by Szczeklik and his colleagues in 1979[5]. In this series, the prostacyclin was given by femoral artery cannulation. In a double-blind controlled trial, 14 patients were randomised to receive a 72-hour intra-arterial infusion of prostacyclin dissolved in glycine buffer and 16 control patients received glycine buffer alone. The starting dose of prostacyclin was 2.5 ng/kg/min, increasing over three hours to 5 ng/kg/min. Patients were assessed before treatment and at 24 hours, 4 weeks and 6 weeks after infusion. By the sixth week, 7 of 21 initial ulcers were healed in the prostacyclin-treated group, whereas in the placebo group the number of ulcers had increased from 29 to 30. At the beginning of the trial there was no difference in mean ulcer area between the two groups, but at its end the area was significantly smaller in the prostacyclin group. By the sixth week the mean ulcer area decreased in the prostacyclin group but not in the placebo group.

Intra-arterial cannulation should be avoided if possible, particularly in the elderly and confused who may pull out the cannula, and Prentice and his colleagues[6] have demonstrated the effectiveness of intravenous prostacyclin in patients with severe arterial disease causing ischaemic rest pain. In the author's clinic prostacyclin is now routinely given intravenously.

The complications of prostacyclin therapy are hypotension and flushing. Most patients will tolerate between 6 and 8 ng/kg/min and it is our policy to start the infusion at 6 ng/kg/min and then cautiously increase by steps up to a maximum of 10 ng/kg/min[7]. Hourly blood pressure measurements are recorded and the nursing staff are particularly asked to look out for flushing. Should either hypotension or flushing occur, the infusion pump is immediately turned down. In a five-year experience of this form of treatment, we have not encountered any serious complications, though a few patients are completely unable to tolerate intravenous prostacyclin therapy. Most patients have been relieved of rest pain and many ulcers have reduced in size, though no precise follow-up figures are available at present. It is now our policy to give prostacyclin intermittently, for 12 in each 24 hours, for a total of 4 or 5 days. If there is no improvement in rest pain after the first 24 hours, the infusion is stopped. If there is definite improvement in rest pain and some diminution in ulcer size at the end of 5 days treatment, skin grafting is performed on the next available operating list. A further course of prostacyclin is started at operation and continued for the first 3 or 4 post-operative days in order to help the graft to take.

There are no definite guidelines to indicate which ischaemic ulcers are likely to respond to prostacyclin therapy, though our experience in treating patients with severe ischaemic rest pain has indicated that those with diabetes and also those with an ankle:brachial pulse pressure index of less than 0.3 are unlikely to respond[7]. These contraindications are of course the same as those for lumbar sympathectomy, as might be expected from the similarity of action of the two vasodilator methods. It seems reasonable to try the effect of a short course of intravenous prostacyclin on all patients with ischaemic ulceration whose arteries are unsuitable for surgical reconstruction (apart, of course, from those mentioned above), or where the patient is unfit for direct arterial surgery and in whom chemical sympathectomy has failed to produce an adequate response. Theoretically prostacyclin should produce no further improvement in a patient who has undergone lumbar sympathectomy, but in practice we have sometimes found it useful.

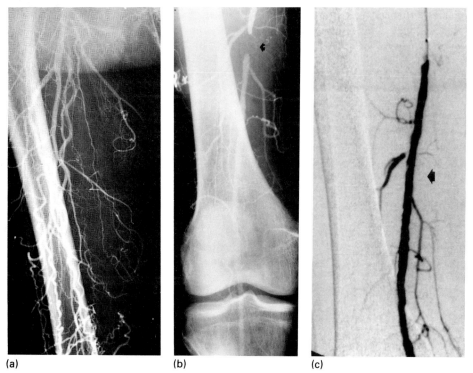

(a)   (b)   (c)

Figure 11.1 Patterns of femoral artery occlusion. (a) Full length occlusion, requires femoropopliteal bypass. (b) Short occlusion, suitable for balloon angioplasty. (c) Following successful angioplasty

Operative surgery and angioplasty

If the popliteal pulse is absent, arteriography should be performed, even in those patients considered unfit for direct arterial surgery, in the hope that the arteriogram will demonstrate a short (less than 10 cm) occlusion of the superficial femoral artery suitable for balloon angioplasty (Figure 11.1b, c). Longer occlusions require treatment by direct arterial surgery. Aortoiliac occlusions are treated by aorto-bifemoral grafting, using a Dacron graft. The modern soft woven grafts are easy to handle and there is no evidence that their patency rate is less than that of knitted grafts. Short occlusions of the superficial femoral artery are best treated by percutaneous transluminal angioplasty (PTA) but long occlusions (Figure 11.1a) will require the insertion of a femoropopliteal bypass graft, using reversed autogenous saphenous vein if possible or, if this is absent or inadequate, a 6 mm PTFE graft. Where the popliteal artery is also occluded, femorocrural graft is then required, preferably using *in situ* saphenous vein, the smaller end of the vein being anastomosed to the smaller artery. In this operation, the valves of the saphenous vein are rendered incompetent by means of a Hall's valvulotome, or similar instrument, and tributary veins are ligated to prevent subcutaneous arteriovenous fistula formation, which can result in painful ischaemic skin necrosis.

Arteriography and arterial surgery in the ulcerated limb: risk of infection

Ulceration adds an extra dimension to the management of the ischaemic limb and must be taken into careful consideration. It is important that the radiologist knows which leg is ulcerated before performing transfemoral arteriography. The opposite femoral artery must always be cannulated. Insertion of a needle or cannula through infected inguinal lymph nodes is likely to result in septicaemia. Care must also be taken in the use of any prosthetic grafts. Ascending infection from an ulcer is likely to cause graft infection, which may prove fatal. It is important therefore that infection is thoroughly controlled before operation, particularly if it is anticipated that a prosthetic graft will be required. This may mean amputating infected ischaemic toes a few days before the arterial reconstruction, or thorough débridement of infected leg ulcers, removing all necrotic tissue down to deep fascia. These procedures are followed by antiseptic dressings and effective doses of the appropriate antibiotics, which are continued during and after arterial surgery. The amputation sites of infected gangrenous toes should be closed loosely over flavine packs at the first operation, secondary closure being delayed until after the effective revascularisation. Similarly ulcers can be grafted, either at the time of the arterial reconstruction or after the reappearance of healthy granulation tissue.

Many patients have a combination of main and small vessel disease and combined treatment may then be necessary, usually by chemical lumbar sympathectomy followed by direct arterial surgery. Chemical lumbar sympathectomy can also improve the blood supply to infected ischaemic ulcers sufficiently to allow antibiotics and local antiseptic cleaning and dressings to remove infection and it should always be considered in the pre-operative preparation of a patient with ischaemic ulceration requiring direct arterial surgery.

Ulceration of mixed arterial and venous origin

The principles of treatment are, not unsurprisingly, exactly the same as those of treating ischaemic ulcers and venous ulcers. Successful management does depend, however, on observing certain priorities. In general, it is important to treat the arterial lesion before attempting any venous surgery, as the incisions required for the latter are unlikely to heal in the absence of a good arterial supply. Caution must be observed in this respect, as direct arterial surgery is inadvisable in the presence of an infected ulcer and is absolutely containdicated if any synthetic graft is required. Fortunately, many patients with mixed arterial and venous ulcers have a short arterial occlusion suitable for balloon angioplasty. If arterial reconstruction is necessary, it is most important to heal the ulcer before this is attempted; however the firm compression required to control venous reflux is likely to exacerbate the ischaemia and therefore lead to ulcer deterioration rather than healing.

These contradictory problems are best dealt with by making every attempt to improve the arterial circulation by non-surgical means before embarking on either arterial or venous surgery. Chemical lumbar sympathectomy alone may be sufficient, but if this is inadequate, a course of intravenous prostacyclin should be tried. This requires admission to hospital and therefore, at the same time as prostacyclin treatment, the ulcer can be treated by light compression bandaging, cleaning and dressings, with appropriate antibiotic therapy. Trental, 400 mg t.d.s., may help in achieving ulcer healing.

If, in spite of these measures, the ulcer is still incompletely healed and arteriograms have shown arterial occlusion requiring bypass surgery, the ulcer should be excised down to deep fascia two or three days before operation, as has been described in the treatment of ischaemic ulcers. Appropriate antibiotics are continued in high doses. Following successful restoration of arterial supply, firm compression bandaging can be applied and venous surgery undertaken in the usual way.

It is the author's experience that, in most of these patients, arterial insufficiency is not severe and very often responds to conservative measures (chemical sympathectomy or prostacyclin), without involving the need for direct arterial surgery. The situation is then not as complicated as might at first appear.

Case report
An overweight young Arab soldier presented with a two-year history of left ankle ulceration which had followed a comminuted fracture of the ankle. Examination showed an ankle venous flare and Doppler ultrasound examination demonstrated calf perforating vein incompetence. The dorsalis pedis pulse was easily felt, but the posterior tibial pulse was impalpable. His foot was warm and apparently well perfused and it was at first thought that the difficulty in finding the posterior tibial pulse was due to ankle oedema. However, Doppler ultrasound examination also failed to demonstrate a pulse and an arteriogram showed that the posterior tibial artery was occluded above the ankle, presumably as a result of the injury.

The patient was treated by chemical lumbar sympathectomy followed by operation to divide and ligate the incompetent perforating vein and graft the ulcer at the same time. The ulcer was healed when he was last seen before his return home.

Amputation

Only too often, arteriography demonstrates very severely diseased arteries, with multiple stenoses and occlusions and very poor, or absent, run-off arteries. The only possible treatment then is chemical sympathectomy or prostacyclin therapy and, if these are ineffectual, continued dressings or amputation are the only remaining options. It is surprising that many patients with ischaemic ulceration experience remarkably little pain, either in the ulcer or in the foot of the affected leg, and prefer to continue with dressings. When however ulceration is accompanied by severe pain requiring continuous analgesics, the patient should be persuaded that amputation is inevitable. A below-knee amputation provides a better functioning limb, but if the blood supply at this level is doubtful, above-knee amputation should be performed in order to ensure good healing and rapid mobilisation of the patient. Prostacyclin infusion pre- and post-operatively will sometimes effect healing of toe or forefoot amputation in patients with proximal arterial occlusion[7], but such limited surgery is more usually reserved for those with diabetic microangiopathy.

Arteriovenous fistulae and venous malformations

Ulcers resulting from arteriovenous fistula formation will only heal if the fistula is effectively closed. Solitary arteriovenous fistulae may be traumatic in origin or may occasionally follow arteriovenous fistulae formation for renal dialysis or femoropopliteal bypass surgery using *in situ* saphenous vein, with inadequate ligation of tributaries. The treatment of solitary arteriovenous fistulae is usually not difficult. They can easily be located by the overlying bruit, helped by arteriography if this is felt necessary, and surgically divided and ligated. Congenital multiple arteriovenous fistulae are more difficult to treat. If relatively localised, e.g. to the palm of the hand, careful dissection under tourniquet with demonstration of the fistulous communications may be possible. The fistulae are ligated and dilated veins excised. More diffuse arteriovenous fistulae, involving a larger area, such as the whole lower limb, are now best treated by a radiologist skilled in therapeutic embolisation. Very severe cases of diffuse fistulae formation may resist all attempts at treatment and require amputation.

Surgery is rarely performed for the Klippel–Trenaunay syndrome, as the diffuse nature of the venous abnormality results in a high incidence of recurrence. Ulceration is not common in this condition and, when it does occur, may respond to firm (Class 1 or 2) elastic compression stockings. If these are ineffectual, surgical treatment may be necessary. It is important to undertake thorough investigation by venograms and varicograms before operation, as some of these patients may have absent deep veins and removal of the superficial veins will then result in intolerable oedema of the limb. Ascending venography must therefore be performed to demonstrate that the deep system is intact. Following this, varicograms are helpful in demonstrating the communication of the varicose superficial veins with the deep system. These abnormal varices are usually most common on the lateral surface of the thigh but their communication with the deep system may be variable. In one of the author's cases, communication with the deep system was through the saphenofemoral junction by way of an abnormally dilated anterolateral vein of the thigh. In another, the communication was with the profunda femoris vein. As in all other surgery of the superficial veins, the surgeon's aim should be to identify and ligate the 'leak point', where the superficial veins communicate with the deep, and avulse individual varices at the same time. The patient must be warned that some varices may recur and that a firm elastic compression stocking must be worn during waking hours during the rest of the patient's life. Careful surgery, followed if necessary by injection sclerotherapy, can result in satisfactory ulcer healing, as has been described in Chapter 8 (page 95).

Contact dermatitis

It is not uncommon to see patients in a leg ulcer clinic whose ulcers are iatrogenic, resulting from medicated bandages or dressings or from the use of local antibiotics. The mainstay of treatment is to stop all such treatment and to substitute bandages or dressings less likely to cause sensitivity. Common causative agents are the rubber in elastic bandages or stockings. Stockings containing Lycra can usually be substituted. Impregnated bandages or dressings may also produce dermatitis; simple non-adhesive Terylene dressings and sterile gauze pads must be substituted. The patient should be referred to the skin clinic for patch testing and any other treatment which a dermatologist may consider helpful.

Rheumatoid and other vasculitic ulcers

Rheumatoid ulcers are extraordinarily difficult to treat. Stacey-Clear and his colleagues[8] have described encouraging results following a course of intermittent intravenous prostacyclin. The author's experience with this treatment has been less encouraging. Active rheumatoid arthritis is usually treated by steroids and the combination of rheumatoid vasculitis and steroid treatment makes any attempt at permanent ulcer healing hopeless. Dressings and bandaging, with control of infection by antibiotics if necessary, is usually all that can be managed in such a situation. When the active disease has become 'burnt-out', treatment by skin grafting can be undertaken with greater hope of success. It is very important to be careful to exclude ischaemia in patients with rheumatoid arthritis. Arteriograms performed in patients referred to the author's clinic with apparently uncomplicated rheumatoid ulcers frequently demonstrate multiple arterial stenoses and occlusions which are not suitable for direct arterial surgery. Amputation may then be the only possible option.

Vasculitic ulcers resulting from other collagen disorders can only be treated conservatively and their healing depends on the course of the underlying disease. Intravenous prostacyclin can be tried, but at present there is no good evidence for its effectiveness.

Steroid ulcers

These will usually heal satisfactorily when the patient can be weaned off steroids. If this is impossible, those physicians responsible for the patient's general management must be asked to reduce steroid dosage to the lowest possible compatible with controlling symptoms.

Hypertensive ulcers

Martorell describes good results, with pain relief and ulcer healing in four of five of his patients treated by lumbar sympathectomy; the fifth patient, who had very severe hypertension and a small, scarred kidney, died postoperatively. Chemical lumbar sympathectomy would now be the treatment of choice. There have been considerable advances in the pharmacological control of hypertension since

Martorell wrote his paper 40 years ago; hypertensive ulcers are therefore less likely to be seen.

Diabetic ulcers

Again, care must be taken to obtain a precise diagnosis of the underlying cause of these ulcers. While most are the result of a combination of diabetic neuropathy and microangiopathy, in a proportion of patients there will also be atherosclerotic main vessel occlusion. Ankle pulse pressures measured by Doppler ultrasound may well appear within normal limits in diabetic patients, due to the stiffness of the vessel walls, and main vessel occlusions may be overlooked. Arteriography is therefore likely to be necessary.

Neither chemical sympathectomy nor prostacyclin are likely to be helpful in the treatment of diabetic ulceration.

Plantar ulceration in diabetics with normal main vessels will usually respond to careful débridement of necrotic tissue, covered by appropriate antibiotics, followed by meticulous avoidance of pressure. This can be achieved by using a Zoppler felt ring or similar pressure relieving pad made of felt or sorbo rubber. The patient must be warned that healing will inevitably be slow and may take several months or a year. Meticulous attention to foot hygiene is necessary during this period. Atherosclerotic main vessel occlusions should be treated by balloon angioplasty or bypass surgery if possible. Unfortunately many occlusions are in the distal lower leg vessels and are therefore not suitable for conventional femoropopliteal bypass surgery. Saphenous vein bypass from the popliteal artery to the dorsalis pedis artery may sometimes be possible but these cases are rare.

Toe or forefoot amputation may be necessary in those with diabetic microangiopathy but normal main vessels, but if the latter are severely diseased, leg amputation, usually below-knee, may be necessary.

Other neuropathies

Avoidance of pressure is the mainstay of treatment in these unfortunate patients. Venous or arterial abnormalities may co-exist with the neuropathy and the patient must be examined with this in mind. An example was an elderly woman with a long history of muscle wasting due to Charcot–Marie–Tooth disease and with ankle ulceration who was found to have absent ankle pulses. Arteriography showed multiple occlusions of the calf arteries. The ulcers responded well to intravenous prostacyclin followed by pinch grafting.

Traumatic ulceration

Traumatic ulcers will heal with dressings and firm compression bandaging or stockings, provided that the underlying blood vessels are normal. Delayed healing of any traumatic ulcer being treated in an accident and emergency department should be recognised and followed by prompt referral to the vascular clinic.

Extravasation of sclerosant during injection sclerotherapy may produce indolent and painful ulcers which are slow to heal and difficult to treat. Each ulcer must be treated individually, but excision is usually the best course. Small superficial ulcers, which may follow injection of venous telangiectasia (spider veins, flare veins), can be excised and the defect closed by primary suture, leaving a scar only a little longer than that usual for the avulsion of varicose veins. The author encountered this complication on a number of occasions when using a 1% solution of Sclerovein (hydroxypolyethoxydodecan). The ulcers usually healed after a few weeks, leaving a small but ugly irregular scar. This was excised without difficulty under local anaesthetic. All patients undergoing injection sclerotherapy must be warned about the possibility of superficial ulceration before treatment has started and the author's patients accepted the minor additional procedure of scar excision without complaint. Since changing the sclerosing solution from Sclerovein 1% to Scleremo (glyceryl chromate) three years ago, no further ulceration has occurred.

Much more serious are those ulcers which may occasionally follow the injection of varicose veins with STD (sodium tetradecyl sulphate). These are usually much larger and more indolent than those following the injection of superficial telangiectasia, and may require treatment by excision and skin grafting. Litigation is liable to ensue, particularly if the patient is an actress or model. In this situation, prevention is clearly better than cure and extreme precautions must always be taken during injection sclerotherapy. Smaller varices are much more safely treated by avulsion under local anaesthetic.

Factitious ulceration

This can be extremely difficult to treat. It is often suspected that a patient may be interfering with the dressings and retarding ulcer healing, but this is usually impossible to prove. Probably the only way of dealing with the situation is to apply a plaster of Paris cast. Even then, patients have been known to poke knitting needles or similar instruments down the plaster cast and continue doing damage to the ulcer surface.

Lymphoedema ulcers

Ulceration is extremely uncommon in lymphoedema and will usually respond to firm compression bandaging or stockings. As has been described, arterial insufficiency can co-exist with lymphoedema and the only patient with ulceration of a lymphoedematous limb who has presented to the author's clinic in recent years was found to have peripheral ischaemia, which was treated by chemical sympathectomy. The combination of lymphoedema and ischaemia is extremely difficult to manage as lymphoedema requires firm compression which, of course, is contraindicated in ischaemia. The ulceration which occasionally occurs in severely oedematous limbs in patients with congestive cardiac failure requires standard conventional treatment by dressings and firm bandaging, with control of the cardiac failure by diuretics and other appropriate drug treatment.

Tropical sores

Initial surgical débridement is usually necessary and this should be followed by full doses of appropriate antibiotics. Unfortunately, the expense involved in poor countries means that quite inadequate courses of these antibiotics are usually prescribed, at least in the Gambia[9]. Macgraith[10] recommends occlusive dressings and bandages which are changed every two or three weeks and may be kept in place by a plaster of Paris cast. Landra[11] argues that, although some ulcers heal, this takes a long time and leaves an unstable scar. He therefore advises excision and grafting of most tropical ulcers. Where the ulcer is complicated by osteomyelitis, lymphoedema or a stiff ankle joint, a below-knee amputation is usually the most practical and economical solution.

Other infectious ulcers

Management is based on appropriate antibiotic treatment of the causative organism, with dressings and bandaging of the ulcer.

Osteomyelitis

This subject is better dealt with in orthopaedic textbooks. Treatment is by rest and long-term antibiotics, with or without exploration of the sinus and drilling or guttering of the bone, as indicated.

Malignant ulcers

Squamous carcinoma

Treatment should be carried out jointly by the surgeon and oncologist and pre-operative assessment of the regional lymph nodes must be undertaken by computerised tomographic scan or lymphography. A small localised squamous carcinoma may be treatable by radiotherapy, but a larger lesion, presenting as a leg ulcer, is more likely to require wide excision and skin grafting. Very large lesions, or where the tumour has penetrated to involve bone, are likely to require amputation. Involved inguinal and iliac lymph nodes will require extensive block dissection followed by radiotherapy.

Basal cell carcinoma

These skin tumours are less likely to present as leg ulcers than squamous carcinomas. Treatment is by surgery or radiotherapy.

Sarcomas

Kaposi's sarcoma and other sarcomas and lymphomas require treatment by surgery, usually amputation, and radiotherapy.

Blood dyscrasias

Simple haematological investigations in the ulcer clinic should demonstrate such conditions as thrombocytopenia, polycythaemia rubra vera and leukaemia. Treatment should be undertaken by a haematologist. Treatment options include aspirin to reduce platelet adhesiveness, venesection for polycythaemia and ^{32}P to produce bone marrow suppression.

Nutritional ulceration

Clearly the ideal solution is to correct the malnutrition at the same time as undertaking simple local treatment of the ulcer. Unfortunately this may not be possible in impoverished societies or in prisoner of war camps. Zinc deficiency can be corrected by appropriate supplements but, as has been discussed above, zinc deficiency seems to be extraordinarily uncommon in the UK, even in elderly patients on low incomes.

Recurrent ulceration

Prevention

All patients with healed ulceration of the legs, whether this is venous or arterial in origin, or from some other cause, are liable to experience a recurrence. Previously ulcerated skin is never as stable as normal skin and care must be taken to prevent even minor trauma. The value of compression hosiery in preventing ulcer recurrence following perforating vein ligation in patients with deep vein incompetence has already been discussed. In addition, some patients without deep vein incompetence also require compression hosiery to protect fragile healed skin at the site of the original ulcers. Deep vein thrombosis must be prevented by the methods outlined in the Appendix. Patients with healed ischaemic ulcers must similarly be careful to avoid trauma and, unfortunately, these patients, who are often elderly and whose eyesight may not be as good as it once was, have an unfortunate tendency to bump into things, particularly supermarket trolleys. On a few occasions, the author has even advised such patients to buy hockey shin pads from their local sports shop and to wear these whenever they go shopping. The heels of bedridden patients with lower limb ischaemia must be protected from pressure by sheepskin or (less expensively) by water-filled surgical rubber gloves under the ankles.

Extremes of heat and cold should also be avoided in patients with healed ulcers. Some years ago, a patient came to the clinic, during a particularly cold winter, with recurrent ulceration of both ankles. Two years previously she had been successfully treated for ankle ulceration by ligation of incompetent perforating veins. She stated that her ulcers recurred after she had waited at a bus stop for over an hour with snow seeping down inside her boots. Careful examination by Doppler ultrasound showed no evidence of further perforating vein incompetence or of popliteal incompetence. Ankle pulses were normal and it was concluded that her recurrent ulcers were simply the result of exposing unstable skin to extreme cold. These ulcers healed successfully with conventional dressings and compression bandaging and with advice to keep warm and avoid waiting at bus stops in the snow.

Investigation and treatment

When a patient presents again in an ulcer clinic, months or sometimes years after appropriate venous or arterial surgery has achieved initial ulcer healing, there is a

Diagnosis and treatment of ischaemic ulceration (1)

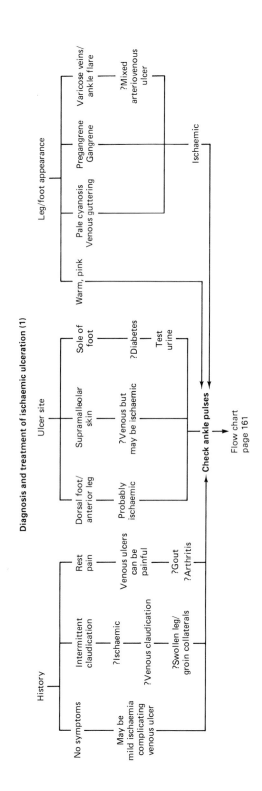

161

Diagnosis and treatment of ischaemic ulceration (2)

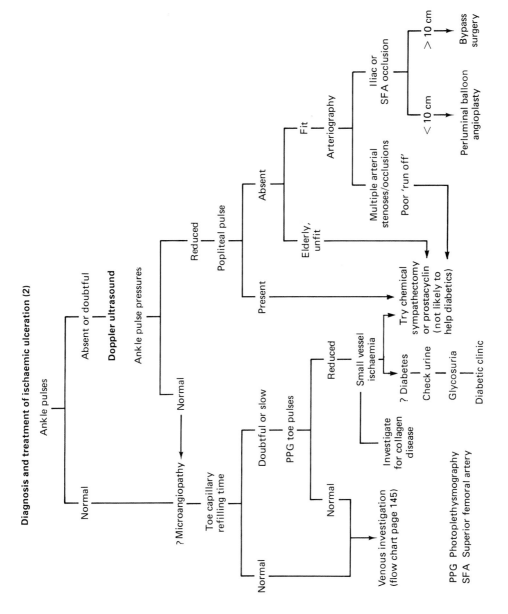

natural tendency to consider the situation hopeless and that conservative treatment by dressings or bandages can be the only form of management in the future. While this may be correct in the very elderly or debilitated patient, who is clearly not fit for any further active treatment, such a pessimistic view should be resisted in the majority of patients presenting with recurrent ulceration. A positive approach must be taken to examination and investigations with a view to finding out the underlying cause of the recurrent ulcer. In the case of a venous ulcer, one or more points of venous incompetence may have been overlooked at the first operation or, alternatively, the responsible vein may have become incompetent since the first operation was performed. The post-malleolar perforating vein may easily be overlooked. Careful examination and investigation by PPG, Doppler ultrasound and venography will often demonstrate a correctable lesion which can be effectively dealt with by further surgery or injection sclerotherapy. In the investigation of recurrent varicose veins, varicography, in which the contrast medium is injected into a varicosity rather than into a dorsal foot vein, is invaluable in demonstrating points of communication ('leak points') between varicose superficial veins and the deep system. Incompetent thigh (hunterian) perforating veins are often responsible for recurrent varicose veins.

In patients with recurrent ulceration and deep venous incompetence, and where no perforating vein or saphenous reflux can be demonstrated, it is worth considering measuring pressures in the long saphenous vein distal to the medial malleolus and, if temporary occlusion reduces the peak systolic pressures produced by calf muscle contraction, ligating the distal long saphenous vein in order to interrupt the pathway for the transmission of high deep venous pressures to the ankle flare veins. An apparently recurrent venous ulcer may in fact be the result of ischaemia due to atherosclerosis which has progressed to arterial occlusion since the original operation for venous incompetence was performed. Ankle pulses must always therefore be carefully examined and followed up by Doppler ultrasound measurement of pulse pressures and arteriography where there is any doubt. Recurrent ischaemic ulceration may result from occlusion of the original bypass graft or from further atherosclerotic stenoses or occlusions in the limb vessels. Intravenous digital subtraction angiography, if available, is a rapid and relatively non-invasive method of investigating such cases. If no other cause for recurrence can be found, consider the possibility of allergy to compression stockings, usually a rubber allergy, and change these to stockings containing Lycra or other synthetic material.

To date, no method of treatment of leg ulcers has ever achieved 100% success, whatever the underlying cause. The surgeon with a busy ulcer clinic is therefore bound to meet many disappointments. However, an optimistic view and a willingness to re-examine and re-investigate apparently hopeless cases will often produce a successful result.

References

1. Moore, W. S., Hall, A. D. Effects of lumbar sympathectomy on skin capillary blood flow in arterial occlusive disease. *J. Surg. Res.* **14**: 151–157, 1973
2. Bracale, G. Is there a place for lumbar sympathectomy for critical ischaemia? In *Limb Salvage and Amputation for Vascular Disease* (eds Greenhalgh, R. M., Jamieson, C. W., Nicolaides, A. N.), Philadelphia, Saunders, 241–255, 1988

3. Yao, S. T., Bergan, J. J. Predictability of vascular reactivity relative to sympathetic ablations. *Arch. Surg.* **107**: 676–680, 1973

4. Linton, R. R. The post-thrombotic ulceration of the lower extremities; its aetiology and surgical treatment. *Ann. Surg.* **138**: 415–430, 1953

5. Szczeklik, A., Nizankowski, R., Skawinski, S., Szczeklik, J., Gluszko, P., Gryglewski, R. J. Successful therapy of advanced arteriosclerosis obliterans with prostacyclin. *Lancet* **1**: 1111–1114, 1979

6. Prentice, C. R. M., Belch, J. J. F., McKay, A. *et al*. Prostacyclin in severe arterial disease. In *Prostacyclin – Clinical Trials* (eds Gryglewski, R. J. *et al.*), New York, Raven Press, pp. 1–5. 1985

7. Negus, D., Irving, J. D., Friedgood, A. Intra-arterial prostacyclin in the management of advanced atherosclerotic lower limb ischaemia. In *Prostacyclin – Clinical trials* (eds Grylglewski, R. J. *et al.*), New York, Raven Press, pp. 107–113, 1985

8. Stacey-Clear, A., Cornwall, J. V., Lewis, J. D. Intravenous Prostacyclin (PGI$_2$) and skin grafting for rheumatoid leg ulcers. In *Phlebology '85* (eds Negus, D., Jantet, G.), London, Libbey, p. 624, 1986

9. Steel, J. R. Personal communication, 1990

10. Macgraith, B. *Exotic Diseases in Practice,* London, Heinemann, 1965

11. Landra, A. D. The tropical ulcer. *Surgery* **59**: 1402–1403, 1988

Chapter 12

Compression hosiery

Compression hosiery is used to control oedema from any cause, to compress varicose veins and to prevent venous thrombosis. This account will concentrate on its role in the prevention and treatment of venous ulceration. It is important that those doctors responsible for running ulcer clinics have some knowledge of elastic hosiery construction and compression values and of the various products available, as this aspect of management is as important as accurate diagnosis and surgical treatment.

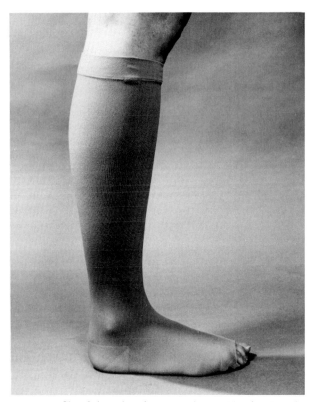

Figure 12.1 Class 2, knee-length compression stocking (Medi UK)

There have been a number of important developments in the design and manufacture of elastic compression hosiery in recent years. Modern garments are better fitted, more comfortable and more effective than those available ten or fifteen years ago (Figure 12.1). Most modern elastic hosiery is of two-way stretch construction, using Lycra for the elastic fibres, though a few manufacturers still use natural rubber. In 1985, a British Standard (BS 6612:1985[1]) was introduced. This was prepared by the Textile and Clothing Standards Committee, which included physicians, surgeons and hosiery manufacturers. The major requirements of the British Standard have been incorporated in a revised Drug Tariff, which now makes it possible for doctors and surgeons to prescribe effective, comfortable and attractive stockings without difficulty.

Stocking pressures and testing methods

The British Standard allows manufacturers to assign a standard compression value (in millimetres of mercury) to each garment, after it has been washed and conditioned for at least sixteen hours in a standard atmosphere. Compression must be graduated up the stocking, from a maximum at the ankle to a minimum at the thigh; the greater the compression at the ankle, the steeper this decrease must be. The standard also specifies the stiffness and durability of garments and requires them to be marked with size, compression value, washing instructions, the manufacturer's label and 'BS 6612:1985'. Stockings in the Drug Tariff are graded into three classes according to the compression they exert at the ankle: Class 1, light (14–17 mmHg); Class 2, medium (18–24 mmHg); and Class 3, strong (25–35 mmHg).

Unfortunately there is still some confusion about measuring stocking pressures as accepted methods vary from one country to another. While all British-made stockings are expected to comply with the Drug Tariff specification and British Standard, with pressures measured by the Hosiery and Allied Trades Retail Association (HATRA) device, there are many excellent brands of stockings available in the UK which are manufactured in Europe, mainly in Germany or Switzerland. German stockings are tested at the Hohenstein Institute by their method, and Swiss stockings by the EMPA test. Details of the HATRA and Hohenstein test methods are given below and the results provided by these two methods are compared. Some stockings are also imported from the USA, particularly by the Kendall Company, and the pressures of these are measured by yet another device, the Instron Tester, a modified tensiometer, which measures the tension in a section of stocking held between two movable T-pins. Stockings tested only by the Hohenstein or EMPA methods have been available for use in hospitals for several years and continue to be so.

These testing devices are all independent of the actual leg on which the stocking is to be fitted. There are devices now available which measure the actual pressure exerted by a compression stocking on the human leg. The first of these was developed by Dr Sigg of Switzerland over twenty years ago. This consisted of a small balloon connected to an aneroid manometer. The balloon is slid under the stocking and the subsequent pressure noted on the manometer. Unfortunately, the shape of the balloon distorts the radius of curvature of the leg and therefore does not measure the pressure accurately. A more recent advance on this device is the Borgnis medical stocking tester (Figure 12.2) which consists of a thin plastic sleeve inserted between the stocking and the leg. Electrodes are printed into the walls of

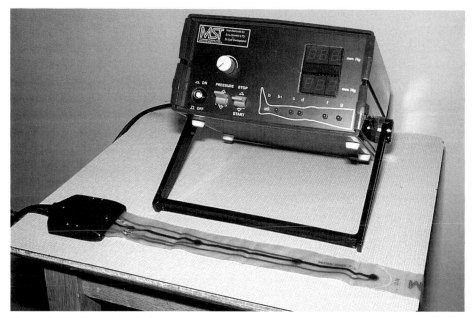

Figure 12.2 The Borgnis medical stocking tester

the sleeve and compressed air is pumped into the sleeve by a small pump. As soon as the pressure produced by the compressed air inside the sleeve overcomes the pressure of the stocking compressing the sleeve against the leg, the proximal pair of electrodes (where the pressure should be least) are forced apart. This breaks an electrical circuit, which automatically stops the pump and simultaneously records the pressure within the sleeve. The pressure is noted and the pump restarted; the pressure increases and provided the stocking is correctly graduated, the next more distal pair of electrodes are then forced apart, stopping the machine and recording the pressure again. This process is continued until all the electrodes in the sleeve have been forced apart and a record of pressures at 10 cm intervals along the leg is then obtained. Care must be taken that the sleeve is not placed over any bony points, which will provide a false reading. This is a simple device and useful for the clinician, who can check that his patients are being fitted correctly by surgical fitters. The disadvantage is that pressures are measured at fixed points and also that the device cannot be left on the leg under a stocking or bandage for any length of time in order to enable serial measurements to be carried out. An advance on the Borgnis tester is the Oxford Pressure Monitor marketed by Talley Medical Limited. The sensors can be placed independently over areas of specific interest and the small plastic sleeves can be retained under compression hosiery for hours or days in order to allow repeat measurements.

HATRA and Hohenstein pressure measurement
The HATRA tester consists of a 'leg former' (Figure 12.3), on which the stocking is placed and then stretched by pulling out a movable bar. A measuring head is then applied to the stretched stocking to obtain the fabric tension at the desired position. The HATRA tester thus requires the stocking to be stretched so that it is in a

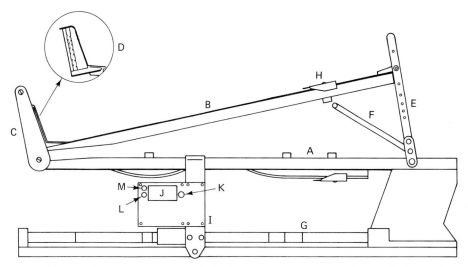

Figure 12.3 The HATRA stocking tester. A, fixed lower bar; B, movable top bar; C, fixed outer foot; D, movable inner foot with adjustment holes; E, upper adjustment bar; F, raising bar; G, traverse rail; H, suspender clip; I, measurement head; J, digital display; K, operating switch button; L, zero adjustment; M, scale adjustment. (Segar Design, Nottingham)

similar energy state to that when it is applied to the leg, whereas the Hohenstein (and the Swiss EMPA) tester tests the stocking in a non-extended form. The Hohenstein tester measures the tension between numerous points marked on a stocking stretched over an expandable leg former by means of a computerised device.

Comparative pressures are illustrated in Figure 12.4, which illustrates that the pressures recorded by the Hohenstein method (and also the EMPA method) are

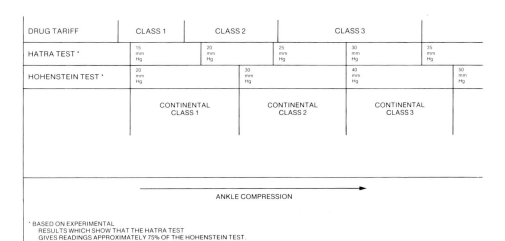

Figure 12.4 The Drug Tariff classification of stocking pressures with HATRA and Hohenstein measurements. Note that the latter are consistently higher in each class

generally higher than those recorded by the HATRA method. The HATRA method also compares better with the (*in vivo*) Borgnis medical stocking tester than the Hohenstein method, and probably therefore gives a more accurate figure of the pressure actually exerted on the leg by the stocking.

Effect on the venous pump

In the following paragraphs, stocking pressures are those measured by the HATRA method, except where otherwise indicated.

Struckmann[2] has demonstrated that venous muscle pump function (assessed by ambulatory calf volume strain gauge plethysmography) in patients with saphenous and perforating vein incompetence is improved by Class 2 and 3 graduated compression stockings exerting pressures of between 20 and 40 mmHg (Borgnis MST) at the ankle. Class 3, 'strong' stockings, providing compression of 25–35 mmHg, have been demonstrated to be effective in improving calf muscle pump function in patients with post-thrombotic deep venous reflux[3]. In practice, Class 2 compression stockings (18–24 mmHg) seem to be equally effective. The precise compression required remains controversial, but it is generally agreed that the hosiery need exert less compression than that theoretically expected from measurements of the ankle venous pressures in patients with superficial or deep venous pathology. During walking, venous pressure at the ankle is about 25 mmHg in normal subjects, 40 mmHg in patients with superficial varicose veins and 60 mmHg in those with post-thrombotic deep vein incompetence. However, hosiery pressures lower than these are effective in controlling oedema and 'heaviness' of the leg and this appears to be for two reasons. Firstly, by Laplace's formula for tubes ($P = T/R$, where P is the pressure in dynes/cm^2, T is the tension in dynes/cm and R is the radius of curvature of the surface being compressed), the pressure exerted on an individual superficial vein with its small radius will be greater than that exerted on the limb as a whole[4]. Secondly, the plasma protein osmotic pressure of 25 mmHg opposes tissue fluid formation and oedema.

Practical applications

Class 1, light (14–17 mmHg) stockings are recommended for simple varicose veins. In fact, simple varicose veins can often be controlled perfectly adequately by lighter hosiery providing only 5–10 mmHg compression. This is due to the Laplace relationship. Most women nowadays prefer wearing tights and, if prescribed on an FP10, these will not be reimbursed by the Family Health Services Authority. Present prescribing regulations treat each leg of a pair of tights prescribed in hospital as a separate prescription item; the present (1991) prescription charge is £3.05; the total cost to the patient is therefore £3.05 × 2 = £6.10, which is greater than the retail price of most support tights with low compression values. Perfectly adequate lightweight support tights can be bought from most major chemists and department stores for less than this prescription price, and patients who are not exempt from paying prescription charges for any reason (old age, unemployment, pregnancy, etc.) are best advised to buy their compression tights without prescription.

In the venous ulcer clinic, the most commonly prescribed stockings are Class 2 (medium) graduated compression stockings, exerting pressures of 18–24 mmHg (HATRA) at the ankle. These include Medi (Medi UK), Venosan 2000

(Credenhill), Varex (Brevet) and Sigvaris 601 (Ganzoni). Knee-length compression stockings are usually perfectly adequate and are much preferred by men. (A number of manufacturers now produce coloured Class 2 compression socks – grey, blue, brown, black, white – which are much preferred for normal daily wear.) These stockings should be prescribed for patients who have had acute deep vein thrombosis and are likely to develop post-thrombotic incompetence of the deep and perforating veins, leading eventually to ulceration. There is no scientific evidence that application of such stockings does in fact delay the onset of ulceration, but post-thrombotic heaviness and oedema is well-controlled by Class 2 stockings and the author's impression is that the more severe symptoms and signs of the post-thrombotic syndrome, liposclerosis and ulceration, do seem to be delayed.

A number of surgeons recommend the use of Class 2 compression stockings, applied over appropriate non-adherent dressings, in ulcer healing. There is no doubt that stockings maintain their pressure better than bandages, but the disadvantage is that exudate from an ulcer will seep through dressings and stain overlying bandages or stockings. Both can be washed, but bandages can be replaced more cheaply than stockings and for that reason elastocrepe bandages covered by Tubigrip stockinette are used in the author's clinic. Others may find Class 2 compression stockings preferable and, as bandages have to be replaced more frequently than stockings, there is probably little difference in the overall cost of healing an ulcer.

In the author's series of 77 patients with 109 ulcerated legs which has been described, patients with evidence of deep venous incompetence were fitted with knee-length Class 2 compression stockings, following ligation of incompetent perforating and saphenous veins. This regimen has given satisfactory results. Only a very few patients, with very large legs or very severe venous disorders, require Class 3 compression stockings. The Sigvaris 503 or 504 stockings (Ganzoni) have proved very satisfactory. Great care must be taken to exclude any arterial insufficiency before prescribing either Class 2 or Class 3 stockings.

Stocking application

Medium compression or strong stockings (Class 2 or 3) may be difficult to apply, particularly for the elderly. Patients with arthritis of the hands may find stocking application quite impossible. In practice, we have found that most patients can get help from a relative or neighbour. However there are a number of tricks and devices which will help. Most Continental stocking manufacturers provide a nylon or silk sock to help the stocking slide over the foot. Rubber washing-up gloves are of considerable help in obtaining a good grip of the top of the stocking and even elderly patients who thought they would be unable to manage find that they can exert sufficient strength with the help of these. Finally, an ingenious device has been developed in Germany and is marketed by Medi UK Limited. This is called the Medi Valet and consists of a plastic-covered steel frame (Figure 12.5) over which the stocking is stretched. The patient slips the foot and ankle into the opened stocking. The frame is then pulled up the leg, allowing the stocking to slip off in the correct position.

One final tip about applying stockings is most useful if, as happens quite frequently, a stocking is a little too long for the patient's leg. The natural tendency then is for the patient to pull hard on the stocking, so as to remove wrinkles in the lower leg and ankle, and then fold over the stocking top so that it lies just below the

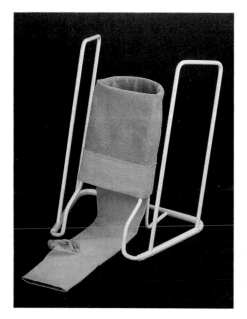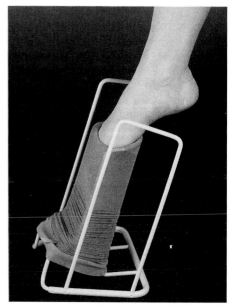

Figure 12.5 The Medi Valet

patella. Folding over the top of the stocking is liable to result in excessive pressure just below the knee with a consequent tourniquet effect, which negates the whole point of a graduated elastic stocking. To avoid this problem the stocking top should be pulled up so that it lies in its natural position just below the patella. If the stocking is a little too long, this will result in wrinkles in the lower leg. Any large wrinkle should be picked up between finger and thumb so that it is converted into two or three smaller wrinkles. These are then rubbed briskly with the hand and, due to the elasticity of the material, they will gradually iron out so that the stocking lies flat and at normal tension. This trick is most useful in practice and I have met few surgical appliance officers, doctors or nurses who were aware of it.

Construction and durability

Until the Drug Tariff was revised in 1988, only rubber elastic threads were permitted in the construction of approved compression hosiery. Rubber is still used and manufacturers of such stockings claim that their elasticity lasts longer than that of stockings made of modern synthetic materials. However, rubber is more susceptible to damage by heat, oil and medicaments and a number of patients become sensitised and develop allergic dermatitis. The new Drug Tariff specification permits the use of Lycra. Most stockings currently available are now of synthetic construction. With wear and tear and regular washing they maintain their elasticity for about three months. It is our policy to prescribe a pair of stockings to any patient with ulceration of one leg. The stockings are interchangeable between legs and they can therefore be worn alternately, one being washed and dried while the other is in use. In this way, a pair should last for six months. It is most important that they are renewed after this time.

References

1. BS 6612 Specification for graduated compression hosiery, Milton Keynes, British Standards Institution, 1985
2. Struckmann, J. Compression stockings and their effect on the venous pump – a comparative study. *Phlebology* **1**: 37–45, 1986
3. Cornwall, J. V., Doré E., Lewis, J. D. To graduate or not? The effect of compression garments on venous refilling time. In *Phlebology '85* (eds Negus, D., Jantet, G.), London, Libbey, pp. 676–678, 1986
4. Fentem, P. H., Goddard, N., Gooden, P. A. The pressure exerted on superficial veins by support hosiery. *J. Physiol.* **263**: 151–152, 1976

The prevention of deep vein thrombosis

As a significant proportion of venous ulcers are the result of deep vein thrombosis and as patients with post-thrombotic deep venous damage have a greater risk of developing further thrombosis when undergoing surgery, it is appropriate to include a brief summary of methods of prevention.

The risk of developing deep vein thrombosis increases with the following factors.

1. A past history of deep vein thrombosis.
2. Age.
3. Malignancy.
4. The contraceptive pill.
5. Major abdominal or thoracic surgery (deep vein thrombosis very rarely follows upper limb, head and neck, or breast surgery).
6. Lower limb fracture or surgery, particularly hip replacement.
7. Obesity.
8. Polycythaemia, thrombocythaemia, hyperfibrinogenaemia and raised blood viscosity.

One hundred and thirty years ago, Rudolph Virchow[1], a German pathologist, described the three major factors responsible for deep vein thrombosis. These are *endothelial damage, stasis* and *changes in coagulability*. Methods of prevention can conveniently be considered under these headings.

Endothelial damage

Fractures or severe soft tissue injury are likely to involve vein trauma and the surgeon cannot do anything about preventing this. Care can however be taken to prevent trauma to the legs during operations by avoiding excessive pressure on the calf muscles. The conventional method of doing this is by putting small padded supports under the ankles; this may prevent trauma to the calf muscles but at the same time is liable to increase stasis due to the suspended muscles hanging flaccidly in a curarised patient. Such ankle supports must therefore be accompanied by compression bandaging or stockings to counteract stasis.

Stasis

Venous stasis in the calf muscle sinusoids, where most deep vein thromboses start, can be counteracted either actively or passively.

Active

Early ambulation must be encouraged. Intermittent calf compression by inflatable plastic leggings[2,3] or by electrical calf muscle stimulation[4] reduces the incidence of ^{125}I-fibrinogen detected thrombi. Neither method has yet been submitted to large scale clinical trial to determine its effectiveness in preventing fatal pulmonary embolism.

Passive

Class 1 compression stockings (Brevet or Kendal TED) reduce the incidence of post-operative deep vein thrombosis by 50%[5] and significantly reduce the incidence of fatal pulmonary embolism[6]. Knee-length stockings are as effective as thigh-length ones[7] and are less expensive, more acceptable to patients and nurses, and are also less liable to roll down and cause a tourniquet effect. The foot of the bed should be elevated post-operatively.

Changes in coagulability

1. Full anticoagulation with warfarin or Dindevan effectively prevents post-operative deep vein thrombosis, but is usually contraindicated after major surgery.
2. Subcutaneous heparin, 5000 units pre-operatively, followed by 5000 units 12-hourly for seven days[8], effectively reduces the incidence of deep vein thrombosis and fatal pulmonary embolism[9], but haematoma at the injection site is quite common and severe post-operative bleeding occasionally occurs[10]. This method should not be used where a significant raw area is left, e.g. prostatectomy, abdominoperineal resection of rectum, etc. It is the method of choice in patients undergoing perforating vein ligation for post-thrombotic ulceration.
3. Low molecular weight dextran, 500 ml during and after operation and 500 ml the following day, is probably less effective in preventing isotope-detected thrombi, but reduces the incidence of fatal pulmonary embolism as effectively as low-dose subcutaneous heparin[11]. The intravenous route is an advantage in patients undergoing thoracic or abdominal surgery, who require intravenous fluids for several days post-operatively. Dextran should be avoided in patients with any impairment of renal function. Acute anaphylaxis has been described, but is extremely rare.
4. An alternative method of prophylaxis in patients requiring intravenous fluids post-operatively is to give intravenous heparin in the very low dose of 1 unit/kg/h (microdose intravenous heparin). This has been demonstrated to reduce the incidence of isotope-detected deep vein thrombosis from 22 to 4%[12]. The heparin must be dissolved in normal saline, which is then 'piggy-backed' into the dextrose infusion line, as it is rapidly denatured in dextrose solution. Ten years experience of this method has shown it to be extremely safe, with no risk of post-operative bleeding or wound haematoma formation.
5. The most recently developed prophylactic agent is low molecular weight heparin analogue. This has been shown to be as effective as heparin in preventing post-operative deep vein thrombosis and carries significantly less risk of bleeding and haematoma formation[13]. It also has the great advantage to patients and nurses of requiring only a once daily injection. Its disadvantage is that at present it is extremely expensive.

The author's policy is to use a combination of the simplest, safest and least expensive mechanical and pharmacological methods. For patients who do not require post-operative intravenous fluid therapy, these are knee-length Class 1 compression stockings, with subcutaneous heparin 5000 units 12-hourly. If low molecular weight heparin becomes less expensive in the future, it will be possible to replace the present 12-hourly injections with a single daily injection. Prophylaxis for patients requiring intravenous fluids consists of knee-length Class 1 compression stockings with intravenous microdose heparin (1 unit/kg/h). This can be simplified to 1000 units 12-hourly except in very light or very heavy patients, in which case the weight-related dose is advisable.

References

1. Virchow, R. *Cellular Pathology as Based upon Physiological and Pathological Histology*, London, Churchill, 1860
2. Sabri, S., Roberts, V. C., *et al.* Prevention of early postoperative deep vein thrombosis by intermittent compression of the leg during surgery. *Br. Med. J.* **4**: 394–396, 1971
3. Hills, N. H., Pflug, J. J., *et al.* Prevention of deep vein thrombosis by intermittent pneumatic compression of the calf. *Br. Med. J.* **1**: 131–135, 1972
4. Browse, N. L., Negus, D. Prevention of post-operative leg vein thrombosis by electrical muscle stimulation. An evaluation with ^{125}I-labelled fibrinogen. *Br. Med. J.* **3**: 615–618, 1970
5. Holford, C. P., Bliss, B. P. The effect of graduated static compression on isotopically diagnosed deep vein thrombosis of the leg. *Br. J. Surg.* **63**: 157, 1976
6. Wilkens, E. R., Mixter, G., Stanton, J. R., *et al.* Elastic stockings in the prevention of pulmonary embolism: a preliminary report. *N. Engl. J. Med.* **246**: 360–364, 1952
7. Porteous, M. J. Le F., Nicholson, E. A., Morris, L. T., James, R., Negus, D. Thigh length versus knee length stockings in the prevention of deep vein thrombosis. *Br. J. Surg.* **76**: 296–297, 1989
8. Kakkar, V. V., Corrigan, T., *et al.* Efficacy of low doses of heparin in prevention of deep vein thrombosis after major surgery. *Lancet* **2**: 101–106, 1972
9. International Multicentre Trial. Prevention of fatal post-operative pulmonary embolism by low doses of heparin. *Lancet* **2**: 45–51, 1975
10. Britton, B. J., Finch, D. R. A., *et al.* Low dose heparin. *Lancet* **2**: 604, 1977
11. Kline, A., Hughes, L. E., *et al.* Dextran 70 in prophylaxis of thromboembolic disease after surgery: a clinically orientated randomised double-blind trial. *Br. Med. J.* **2**: 109–112, 1975
12. Negus, D., Friedgood, A., *et al.* Ultra low dose intravenous heparin in the prevention of post-operative deep vein thrombosis. *Lancet* **1**: 891–894, 1980
13. Kakkar, V. V., Murray, W. J. G. Efficacy and safety of a low molecular weight heparin (CY216) in preventing post-operative venous thrombembolism. In *Phlebology '85* (eds Negus, D., Jantet, G.), London, Libbey, p. 416, 1986

Index